How to Comfort
the Sick and Dying

Rev. Jos. A. Krebs, C.SS.R.

ROMAN CATHOLIC BOOKS
P.O. Box 255
Harrison, NY 10528

Nihil Obstat.

REMY LAFORT,
Censor Librorum.

Imprimatur.

✠ MICHAEL AUGUSTINE,
Archbishop of New York.

NEW YORK, February 22, 1898.

ISBN 0-912141-11-5

TO

Jesus,

HELP OF THE SICK,

Mary,

CONSOLATION OF THE AFFLICTED,

Joseph,

PATRON OF THE DYING,

WITH THE HEARTFELT WISH THAT IT MAY CONDUCE

TO THE SALVATION OF MANY SOULS,

THIS BOOK IS DEDICATED,

IN ALL HUMILITY,

BY THE AUTHOR.

PREFACE.

MANUALS for the sick, containing instructions on the best way of tending and assisting the sick and dying, and of helping them to sanctify sickness and death in a truly Christian manner, are certainly not wanting. But I know of no book expressly destined for *sick-nurses*, and in particular for *religious* who devote themselves to the care of the sick. And yet it is of great importance that they should clearly discern what a sublime and blessed, but at the same time what a difficult, task they have to fulfil, and how they should accomplish it. With this view the present work has been undertaken. It deals in detail with the care of the sick as a vocation, and gives instructions on the best way to render spiritual assistance to the sick and dying.

The book treats only of the spiritual care of the sick and in the sense of the Catholic Church; the care of the body is not included, because it is supposed that the sick-nurses already possess all necessary knowledge of this.

According to the recognized principle that " words instruct, but examples attract," about *one hundred examples,* suitable for the nurses as well as for the sick, have been inserted in the proper places. Care has been taken in the choice of these examples to select only such as are true and are from reliable sources.

In order to render the book a *complete manual* for religious who attend the sick, different prayers and devotional exercises (especially examinations of conscience on the care of the sick) are given in an appendix; by which means the sanctification of their own souls is taken into consideration.

VAALS, HOLLAND,
Feast of the Nativity of Our Lady
September, 1894.

CONTENTS.

PART I.

THE SERVICE OF THE SICK CONSIDERED AS A VOCATION.

8 *Contents.*

FOR THE SICK.

Illness a Medicine.

Illness a Chastisement.

Illness a Touchstone.

Illness a Source of Merits.

Resignation to the Will of God.

Suffering Illness Joyfully.

THE HOLY SACRAMENTS.

Confession.

PART I.

THE SERVICE OF THE SICK CONSIDERED AS A VOCATION.

CHAPTER I.

₩be Service of tbe Sick is a Sublime Wocation.

THERE is a twofold reason for considering the
service of the sick a sublime vocation. First, by it
the commandment of charity is perfectly fulfilled;
and secondly, because our divine Saviour Himself
is served in the person of the sick.

I. BY SERVING THE SICK THE COMMANDMENT OF CHARITY IS FULFILLED IN A MOST PERFECT MANNER.

Illness is generally considered as one of the
greatest temporal evils that can befall man in this
life; it is therefore a great act of loving-kindness,
a work of mercy, to visit the sick, in order to console them and as far as possible to alleviate their

sufferings. The heartfelt sympathy shown to a
sick man is so soothing to him that from it alone
he often derives great relief.

It is well known that the love of our neighbor
is founded on that law of nature which teaches
man to do to others as he would that they should
do to him. Now, since in the time of sickness we
desire nothing more than help and consolation
from others, it is a duty even of the natural law
of charity to endeavor to assist and console our
neighbor to the best of our power. Hence it is
we read in the Old Testament that the three
friends of Job, although heathens, on hearing of
his affliction, came from afar to visit and console
him by their sympathy.

God having thus engraved the commandment of
charity on the heart of man, it is no wonder that
He should have inculcated it in a special manner
in the Old Testament. Thus we read in the Book
of Ecclesiasticus (vii. 39): " Be not slow to visit
the sick, for by these things thou shalt be confirmed in love "—which means, as the commen-
tators of Holy Scripture say, that on the one hand
it furnishes us with occasions for various practices
of charity, and on the other obtains for us the love
of our fellow men. In the New Testament, which
is above all a law of love, our divine Saviour has
taught us by His own example to care for the
sick, and sanctioned it as a duty. " He went
about," says Holy Scripture, " doing good to all ";
nevertheless the sick were especially the objects of
His compassion; "healing," as the Gospel says,

"every disease, and every infirmity" (Matt. ix. 35); "and whithersoever He entered, into towns or into villages or cities, they laid the sick in the streets, and besought Him that they might touch but the hem of His garment, and as many as touched Him were made whole" (Mark vi. 56). Most of the miracles of Our Lord were wrought in favor of the sick, and He willed that His apostles should likewise possess and exercise this gift of miracles on behalf of the sick. And why so? In order to show us His great love and heartfelt sympathy for the sick, and to incite us in like manner to have compassion on them. In this case, as in all the acts of His mortal life, He wished to give us an example, that we might do likewise. All this is confirmed by the express order of Our Saviour when He says: "This is My commandment, that you love one another, as I have loved you" (John xv. 12). He means thereby to say: My love is the measure by which you can learn how you ought to love one another. Even as I have been full of compassion and tenderness towards the sick, so also should you be full of cordial love for them; as I have gone in search of the sick, lavishing on them consolation and help, so also should you render them all the service in your power. It is by this love for your fellow men, and above all for the suffering members of the great human family, that you should be known as My disciples.

This love of the sick was consequently practised in the earliest times of the Church and with the greatest heroism, especially by those pious women

who, according to the Acts of the Apostles, consecrated themselves to the care of the sick and the
poor.   It was not long before regular hospitals
were erected for the sick poor in the larger towns.
St. John Chrysostom opened several at Constanti-
nople, the capital of the Eastern Empire.   Before
this period, Fabiola, a rich Roman widow, had already founded a hospital at Rome.   " She was,"
writes St. Jerome, " the first to open a hospital at
Rome, there to shelter and tend the unfortunate
beings who lay perishing in the streets from poverty and sickness."   He goes on to say how Fabiola
herself used to carry to the hospital invalids attacked with revolting or contagious maladies; how
with her own hands she washed their wounds, gave
them to eat, and, in a word, attended to them
with so much devotedness that many a one in
health was jealous of the poor invalids in the
hospital.

And how many different religious Orders and
Congregations for the service of the sick have
since then sprung up within the Catholic Church !
Who with greater right than they can lay claim to
the perfect accomplishment of the commandment
of charity, according to the words of our divine
Saviour: " Greater love than this no man hath,
that a man lay down his life for his friends " ?
And this is exactly what those religious do who
give themselves up to the service of the sick:
they renounce everything they possess in the
world, in order to become victims of love in the
service of the sick.   By their vow of poverty they

relinquish all earthly goods, to give them to their divine Saviour in the person of the poor. They resign their own will and liberty, in order that, as often as obedience requires, they may tend the sick without intermission all the days of their life. They bid adieu to all sensual pleasures and enjoyments, are ready to sacrifice their health and strength, and to sit day and night near sick-beds or in crowded wards, where they hear nothing but plaintive sighs and groans.

Such disinterested love in these religious wins the admiration even of the children of this world, who in the most critical cases do not hesitate to take advantage of their spirit of self-sacrifice. If some one, for example, be attacked by a repulsive or contagious malady, who is there to nurse him ? Friends and acquaintances ? By no means; fear of becoming a prey to the same illness keeps them from the invalid. Even the nearest relatives often shun the presence of the unfortunate invalid, and in spite of their natural love and attachment they refuse to expose themselves to the risk of assisting him at such a time. Whose courage is so great as to compel him to remain with the invalid in this critical state ? Who will nurse him ? Who will console and assist him day and night ? Who will brave the danger and be ready to sacrifice life for the sake of the poor sufferer ? People in the world know well to whom they must apply in such cases, being fully aware of the noble spirit of self-sacrifice of the Brothers and Sisters of Charity. What they often decline to do themselves for their nearest relatives they expect from religious, who for the love of God and from pure, supernatural love of their neighbor consecrate themselves to the service of the sick, yea, even deem it a happiness to forfeit life in serving them. Every religious Congregation devoted to the service of the sick is prepared to furnish numbers of such martyrs of charity. Let us not wonder, then, that even infidels delight in seeing such heroic sick-nurses at their bedsides and welcome them as consoling angels in human form. Hence it is that the soldier goes to the battle-field with a lighter heart if he knows that in the case of being severely wounded, or otherwise exposed, to the danger of losing his life, the well-skilled hand and the loving care of a Brother or Sister of Charity are ready to succor him.

II. THE SERVICE OF THE SICK IS A SUBLIME VOCATION, BECAUSE THEREBY OUR DIVINE SAVIOUR HIMSELF IS SERVED.

When we see a fellow-creature suffering, ordinary sympathy prompts us to do for him what in a similar situation we would look for on the part of others; that is to say, to hold out to him a helping hand. But Christian charity demands that we should love and assist our neighbor, and above all the sick, even as Christ our Lord taught us by His own example when on earth. Nay, more: our divine Saviour assures us that He will consider every act of charity rendered to the sick as a service to Him; consequently we visit, serve, and console Him in the person of the sufferer. Now, if we hear of some one being ill, we should be as much affected by the news as if we knew Our Saviour Himself to be ill. When about to visit the sick we should represent to ourselves that it is Jesus Christ whom we are going to visit; when we console him, or in any way come to his assistance, let it be with the same tender compassion which we should feel if we were to behold the Son of God in a suffering state.

In order to convince us that this view is not merely imagination, but the pure and simple truth, Our Lord assures us that our final sentence on the last day will depend upon whether or not we have served and succored Him in the person of the poor, the sick, and the suffering. For on that day He will say to the elect standing at His right hand: " Come, ye blessed of My Father, possess ye the kingdom which has been prepared for you from the foundation of the world." As one of the titles to this everlasting bliss, the Lord goes on to say: " I was sick and you visited Me." And to the inquiry of the just: " Lord, when did we see Thee sick and visit Thee ? " He will reply : " Amen I say to you, whatsoever you have done to one of the least of these My brethren, you have done it unto Me."

That exalted model of Christian charity, St. Vincent of Paul, alludes over and over again to this supernatural motive in the conferences addressed to the members of the pious Association which he founded for the relief of the sick. " When we visit the sick," he says, " we find in them everything that is repugnant; but if we regard them in the light of faith, we see in them the image of our sweet Saviour, who makes the sufferings of the poor His own, and who wills that we should honor Him in the person of the poor and afflicted."

If those who consecrate themselves to the care of the sick were not penetrated with this lively faith, we should seek in vain for that spirit of self-sacrifice and that courage which they exhibit in their vocation. Who indeed without this lively faith would bind himself to renounce the world and the prospect of wealth, honors, and pleasures, and consecrate himself without reserve to the Lord, in order to render Him in the person of the sick the lowest services, and that not for a few weeks or months only, but for a whole lifetime, until the very hour of death ?

Our Lord has at various times and in a marvellous manner shown that in reality we wait upon and assist Him in the person of the sick. Thus Pope Leo IX., when still Bishop of Toul, happened one day to meet a poor leper in the street. Taking him to his own house, he washed him, gave him to eat, and laid him in his own bed to rest. After this he locked the room and house and went to attend to his pastoral duties. On his return, when he unlocked the doors to look after his guest, he found that he was gone, from which he concluded that it was Christ our Lord Himself, who had taken the form of a leper in order to put his charity to the test.

St. John Colombini, founder of the Order of the Jesuats, while yet in the world, went one day to assist at holy Mass. At the church door he met a beggar whose whole body was covered with repulsive ulcers. Touched at the sight, John took the sick man in his arms and carried him to his house. There the sufferer was laid in the saint's own bed, and his wife was told to care for the man until his return. In compliance with her husband's wishes, the good woman went at once to the room in which the poor man had been placed, but to her surprise on opening the door a heavenly fragrance was wafted towards her. Filled with a holy fear, she did not dare enter. The saint shortly after returned from church, and they went together to the sick man's bed; but lo ! he had disappeared. A few days later Christ our Lord appeared to St. John and told him that He was the sufferer whom he had so lovingly received.

St. Elizabeth of Hungary, after having washed and cleansed several lepers, wiped them with costly linen, and carefully put them to bed, said to her maids: "How happy are we to be able thus to serve and tend our divine Lord ! " There was no act of charity for the sick which appeared too lowly or too perilous for this holy princess; for in each sufferer she beheld the likeness of her divine Spouse, and to those who inspired her with the greatest repugnance she devoted herself with special tenderness.

A person consecrated to God considers it a privilege to be able to serve the divine Master in the person of the sick. When kneeling at the bedside of the sufferer, she imagines herself to be at the feet of her Saviour, and consequently treats the sick one with as much regard and holy reverence as though she were tending Our Lord Himself. The service of the sick is truly a sublime vocation if considered in the light of faith. It is true that there are few in this world who envy those who are called to such a vocation: but if the angels in heaven were capable of envy, they would undoubtedly covet the lot of those who devote themselves to the service of the sick and are permitted to tend the King of heaven in the person of His suffering members.

CHAPTER II.

The Service of the Sick a Blessed Vocation.

THE service of the sick can be called a blessed vocation because, first, it makes us perform great things for the glory of God; secondly, because we render the most important services to the sick; and thirdly, because we ourselves derive great benefit therefrom.

I. WHEN SERVING THE SICK WE DO GREAT THINGS FOR THE GLORY OF GOD.

1. It is a well-known fact that by training youth to a pious life much can be done for the greater glory of God; but it is evident, also, that much more can be obtained by the infirmarian who, in sanctifying the last days of the sick, brings safely into the storehouse of eternity the fruits of a good education and a Christian life which perhaps, in the course of years, have been stained by sin. Hence it was that St. Francis Regis, that great friend of the sick, used to say: " The good we do among poor sinners in their days of health is exceedingly precarious. We sow the good seed, it is true, but the enemy at the same time sows cockle

so that the good seed is too often choked by it. But the work of mercy which we perform towards the sick and dying is not long exposed to the influence of human frailty, nor are the wiles of Satan, as a rule, able to destroy it, for the dying man generally perseveres in his good dispositions unto the end." If, while serving the sick, we were mindful only of their bodily interests, without considering the salvation of their souls, this charitable work would contribute but little towards the glory of God. Both in body and in soul the sick belong to God; nay, even more in soul than in body, the soul being the principal object of His love. God sends illness to men in order to procure their eternal salvation. In like manner, nursing the sick should be practised so as to further the designs of God and enable the invalid to attain his last end. A good sick-nurse avails himself of every opportunity to speak with the patient on pious subjects, especially of the last truths of religion, reminding him that there is only one thing absolutely necessary—the salvation of his soul. Oh, how many poor sinners, sunk in forgetfulness of God and plunged into all sorts of vices, have been touched by the salutary admonitions of a zealous sick-nurse and brought back to God by true contrition and complete change of life !

2. Moreover, the glory of God is increased in no small degree by the simple fact that there is nothing so much calculated to obtain esteem and confidence for the Holy Catholic Church as the

loving care with which her best and most faithful children devote themselves to the welfare of their sick and dying fellow men. This devotedness is recognized even by men who are cold and indifferent in regard to all that concerns religion. Nay, it is admired even by infidels, and they find in it a more convincing proof of the divine origin of our faith than in the most subtle reasoning, as the godless Voltaire and many others have avowed. When careless Christians witness the indefatigable zeal of a Brother or Sister of Charity in tending the sick; when they see these good religious, day and night, at every hour and season, ready to assist the sick; when they see that neither poverty, nor misery, nor the most revolting maladies alarm them, and that they do all this for God's sake, with no other end in view than the good of the sick, both spiritual and corporal; that in order to accomplish this work of charity they sacrifice their natural inclinations, their rest, their health, and even their lives—this is what fills such lukewarm Christians with admiration, moves them to the very heart, and not unfrequently leads to the most striking conversions. Truths which can be seen and, as it were, handled, are far more convincing than those which come to us through the sense of hearing alone.

3. If the loving care of the sick always makes a favorable impression, much more powerful will be its influence when, in the time of sorrow and mourning, it appears as a consoling angel in the house. How can loving children ever forget the

visits of the angel of charity, who entered their
house day and night to prepare their parents for a
holy death ?   How can they forget that those
hours of bitter bereavement were thus rendered
more endurable ?   Even after the lapse of many
years they will love to tell their friends and relatives how calmly and peacefully their beloved
parents fell asleep in the Lord.   Again, how many
parents there are who have to weep for long years
over some prodigal son hurrying down the way of
perdition.   At length, overcome by the influence
of loving care in time of sickness, the prodigal is
converted; he repents of his sinful ways; his soul
is won for heaven in his last moments.   Oh, with
what heartfelt gratitude will these parents bless
and praise the mercy of God, and how grateful
will they be to the one whom God employed as
His instrument to snatch their child from the
clutch of Satan at the very threshold of eternity !

II. BY NURSING THE SICK THE MOST IMPORTANT SERVICES ARE RENDERED TO THE SICK MAN HIMSELF.

1. A holy death being the greatest of all graces,
and the danger to which the human soul is exposed at the hour of death being likewise the
greatest of all dangers, it is easy to see that we
cannot render a greater charity to our neighbor
than by helping him to die holily.   St. Alphonsus
does not hesitate to assert that there is no work of
mercy more pleasing to God and more profitable

to our neighbor than that of assisting man at the hour of death. Why is this ? " Because," says the holy doctor, " our destiny for all eternity depends on death; at no other time are we exposed to such violent and dangerous temptations as at the approach of death, when hell redoubles its efforts; finally, the sufferer is himself so enfeebled that without extraordinary help he will scarcely be able to resist the attacks of his spiritual enemies." God more than once gave St. Philip Neri to understand how pleasing this act of charity is in His eyes, by showing him the angels, who, while the religious were occupied in nursing the sick, suggested to them the words they were to make use of in order to touch their hearts and give them salutary encouragement in the last moments of their lives.

It is doubtless a generous and highly meritorious act to rescue a person from any imminent danger of fire or shipwreck; the State itself recognizes this, and rewards such an action by a mark of special distinction in testimony of its approval. But he who helps a fellow man to die a happy death does infinitely more and is far more deserving of praise and recompense, not only because he has snatched another from everlasting ruin, but because he has been the means of procuring for him the eternal joys of heaven.

What a happy vocation it is, then, to tend the sick in their bodily necessities with the design of obtaining for them what is of far more importance —the cure and sanctification of their souls and

the enjoyment of everlasting happiness in heaven !
Many sick people under the loving care of religious
have been restored to health; but many more of
those who were spiritually dead, have through the
generous love and devotedness of their nurses been
brought to a new life by a sincere return to God.
For, when the sick man notices the tender care
with which the religious serves him day and night,
and thinks that all this is done not for pay but
simply for the love of God, many an earnest
thought forces itself upon him. He sees himself
so deserted and solitary; his best friends and
nearest relatives evince for him far less affection
and interest than he receives at the hands of
strangers. He plainly sees that those who love
God and their neighbor for God's sake are truly
happy and contented, while he, in the bondage of
sin and a slave to his passions, has forfeited the
grace and friendship of God, and with it inward peace and true happiness. How, then, can
he resist the friendly exhortations to reconcile
himself once more with God: especially as the
words of a benefactor, to whom we are greatly in-
debted, exercise a powerful influence over the
heart ?

In the days of health we but too easily lose sight
of the remembrance of God and the eternal truths.
Business, pleasure, the din and tumult of the
world—all these are but too apt to drive from our
minds the teachings of faith and to stifle the voice
of conscience. But in illness it is very different.
A man confined to his room, and to that bed which

he will, perhaps, never more leave, begins to reflect seriously, and to be more susceptible to the
influence of grace. Then his thoughts turn to
God; he begins to fear His justice, while His
goodness and mercy inspire him still more with
confidence. The infirmarian can find in these
dispositions a favorable opportunity to induce the
sick man to regulate his conscience and to prepare
the way for the priest whose privilege it is to bring
the lost sheep back to its Shepherd.

2. But the activity of a zealous sick-nurse does
not end here; he pursues the work which has been
so happily begun, and accompanies the dying man
to the very gates of eternity. How often are the
sick subject to depression and interior desolation !
How often are they tortured by physical pain, the
sufferings of the present time, as well as those
which they foresee in the future ; perhaps by
the indifference and coldness of those who ought
to show their love and yet do not ! All this is
often a cause of profound sadness to the sick man,
and in this state of dejection he finds nothing to
allay his grief or to raise his drooping spirits. In
these circumstances there is no greater happiness
for him than to find a true friend, a compassionate
and loving consoler in his infirmarian. On the
other hand, what a glorious vocation is that
which makes one in very truth a Brother, a Sister
of Charity, an apostle of Christian love to these
poor sufferers ! In a few days this or that sick
person will no longer be numbered among the
living; he will have entered the eternal home,

and the time of merit for him will be forever
at an end. But during the short interval yet
granted him by God how much he can lose, how
much he can gain for all eternity ! If he is
strengthened by salutary exhortations, pious reading, suitable prayers, and words of encouragement,
he will bear his sufferings with patience and resignation, and by thus sanctifying and rendering
them meritorious he will be enabled to overcome
many violent and dangerous temptations; he will
willingly receive death from the hand of God; in
many cases he will perhaps be purified from even
the smallest faults and offer perfect atonement to
the divine justice, and after a brief purgatory, or
even without passing through purgatory at all,
will go to receive an unfading crown in heaven.

III. THE SICK-NURSE HIMSELF GAINS GREAT PROFIT FROM SERVING THE SICK.

1. First of all, infirmarians by their intercourse
with the sick have many *salutary thoughts* brought
before them. Persons who have to deal continually with the sick are not infrequently deemed
worthy of compassion, because their eyes behold
nothing but misery; yet it is precisely from this
that they derive great advantage. Is it not one
of the greatest evils to esteem too highly this
earthly life and attach our hearts too much to the
things of this world ? The result of this attachment is to cool our zeal for the perfection and salvation of our souls. It is therefore of the greatest

importance that the vanity of all earthly things as well as the depth of human misery should be brought vividly before our eyes. And this is exactly what the service of the sick most frequently forces us to behold. For instance, you are called to the sick-bed of a rich man who but a few days ago was numbered among the happiest of mortals. In possession of a vast fortune, he was honored and esteemed; the choicest gifts of the world were at his command; his happiness seemed supreme. But now suddenly all is changed; all that he formerly possessed and loved serve now only to increase the intensity of his pain; from the summit of human prosperity he will soon descend into the grave and be forgotten. Does not such a sight bring forcibly to your mind the vanity of all earthly things ? Again you are called to the sick-bed of one to whom youth, blooming health, and a strong constitution seemed but a few days before to promise a long life. And behold ! now he lies prostrate at the very verge of the grave. He is consumed by a devouring fever, and owing to a complication of maladies the doctors are unable to do anything for him—in a few hours he will be the prey of death. Does not such a sight forcibly remind the infirmarian of the frailty of life and of the certainty of death ? In the same way the service of the sick suggests many other salutary considerations. The sight of the sinful as well as the pious Christian, of those who have been able to prepare for death, as well as those who are surprised by a sudden death, inspires the sick-nurse with deep and serious reflections. Many a time the justice of God manifests itself in an appalling manner to his view; still oftener he is a witness of the unspeakable patience and mercy of the Lord, leading the wandering sinner to penance and amendment at the end of his earthly career. Some afford him edification by their heroic patience and resignation to the divine will, while in others he can but recognize the avenging arm of God's justice, who, even in this world, chastises man for his iniquities and causes him to feel the bitterness of sin. Oh, how many opportunities there are at the bedside of the sick and dying, not only to consider the truths of religion, but, as it were, to see them with one's own eyes and to touch them with one's own hands !

2. Moreover, attendance upon the sick furnishes an excellent opportunity of *practising many virtues,* and of following the example of our divine Saviour, who was more ready to see and cure the servant of the pagan centurion than the daughter of Jairus, the head of the synagogue. Even so an infirmarian who is animated by the right spirit goes as willingly, nay, even more readily, into the dwellings of the poor than into the sumptuous mansions of the rich, and thus practises the precious virtue of *humility.* Then, again, sick people are generally very capricious, wishing and asking for things that it is often impossible to grant them, and the weakness of the mind surpasses even that of the body. In such cases a good infirmarian arms himself with tender compassion and untiring

meekness. He does not allow himself to be dis-
heartened by their spiritual infirmities, nor to yield
to impatience; he bears with their bad humor,
tries to accommodate himself as far as possible to
their strange fancies, and to gratify their wishes,
provided these are harmless in themselves.

In serving the sick, self-love finds no satisfac-
tion; the whole character of this service, being
repugnant to natural feelings and natural inclinations, calls for the continual exercise of *Christian
mortification.* The many annoyances and troubles which this occupation entails cannot be patiently borne except by a generous self-renunciation, so that the service of the sick may justly be
termed a continual penance. What patience, what
self-denial are necessary to bear the bodily fatigue,
the watching, the natural repugnance, the various
cares, and often in addition to this the rudeness,
the complaints, and the ingratitude of the sick,
and yet not lose courage ! One single week devoted to such a labor of love is productive of more
virtues than whole months spent in bodily austeri-
ties of our own choice.

3. He who zealously devotes himself to the care
of the sick may confidently expect a happy death.
Divines assure us that almsgiving (by which are to
be understood not only gifts in money, but all
works of charity in general) is in a certain way as
necessary to a man to enable him to attain his end
as Baptism is to a new-born infant, since other
good works, such as prayer and fasting, are of no
avail without almsgiving. Thus, for instance,

the Pope St. Leo says : " Let no one flatter
himself on account of his good life if he is deficient in good works." " Wherefore," the prophet
Daniel (iv. 24) says: " Redeem thou thy sins with
alms, and thy iniquities with works of mercy to the
poor." The Holy Ghost in like manner exhorts
us in various places to take great care to practise
works of mercy, because these acts of brotherly
love make us firm, steady, and persevering in the
love of God. " Be not wanting," says Ecclesiasticus (vii. 38, 39), " in comforting them that
weep, and walk with them that mourn. Be not
slow to visit the sick: for by these things thou
shalt be confirmed in love." Thus, steadfastness,
that perseverance in good, the grace of graces,
which the saints prayed for with so many prayers
and sighs, is promised as a reward to the merciful.
Although there are various signs of predestination,
yet compassion for the poor and the oppressed,
and the endeavor to help them in their needs, are
among the most pre-eminent. " Put ye on therefore," says St. Paul (Col. iii. 12), " as the elect of
God, holy, and beloved, the bowels of mercy."
And in the Old Testament the Holy Ghost exhorts us to be compassionate and merciful: " And
thou shalt be as the obedient son of the Most
High, and He will have mercy on thee more than
a mother " (Ecclus. iv. 11).

It is a well-known fact that those who tend the
sick pass out of this world with indescribable tranquillity, God assisting them in the supreme moment and inspiring them with a strong confidence

in His mercy, according to the words of Tobias (iv. 12): " Alms shall be a great confidence before the Most High God, to all them that give it." Therefore St. Peter Chrysologus says: " In vain is he accused by his sins who is excused by the poor." The experience of all ages confirms the words of St. Jerome (*Epist. ad Nepotian*) uttered as early as the fourth century: " I do not remember having seen a man who had done much good to the poor die a bad death." And St. Vincent of Paul asserts that he had often experienced how in their last hour God withdrew the fear of death from the merciful, however much they might have been troubled by it during life. May not a person rightly expect to be assisted in a special manner by God at the hour of death when she has spent a great part, nay, perhaps the greatest part of her life in serving the sick, toiling day and night, and thus sanctifying herself, having perhaps lost her health and shortened her life ? May not such a one, who has been an angel of consolation to so many of her fellow men, confidently hope that in her last hour He will also send her an angel to fill her with heavenly comfort ?

4. If every good religious may justly hope to find in God *a merciful Judge* after death, this must in a special manner be applicable to those who during their lifetime have devoted themselves to the care of the sick. There is no doubt that the judgment will be according to the rules of the strictest justice, extending not merely to an account of the sins, but also of the good works done

during life.   Nevertheless a religious entrusted
with the care of the sick need have no fear of an
unfavorable sentence.   One who at all times is
resolved rather to die than to commit mortal sin
(and we may well presuppose such a disposition in
an infirmarian) may be sure of being in God's
grace, and need not fear to be sentenced to everlasting damnation.   This hope of meeting with a
merciful judgment is confirmed by all that she has
done and suffered in the religious state and especially while serving the sick: the patience and compassion which she has lavished on them, the
mortification she has undergone, the humility with
which she gladly made herself the servant of all,
the many grievous pains she has endured, etc.
How can such a religious fear to appear in the
presence of her Saviour, whom in the person of
the sick she has served so long and so faithfully ?
How can the Lord condemn those who throughout their whole lives have condemned themselves
to so painful a service and to such manifold privations ?   Does not He, the eternal and infallible
Truth, say that He will welcome them with the
consoling words: " I was hungry and you gave Me
to eat; I was thirsty, and you gave Me to drink;
I was sick, and you visited Me: come, good and
faithful servant, enter into the joy of your Lord" ?
They may indeed have many failings to expiate,
many debts to pay to the justice of God; but the
grateful souls to whom they rendered such numerous services will undoubtedly help them to
clear away very speedily the debts.

5. And finally, what a *rich reward* in heaven will be the lot of the faithful infirmarian! God is faithful to His promises. If He has expressly promised to requite even a drink of water given in His name, how richly will He reward those who times without number have presented to the sick not only a glass of water or other refreshing beverage, but who have spent their whole lives in ministering to the corporal and spiritual wants of the sick to the best of their power, lavishing upon them every kind of affectionate interest! The whole life of such a religious has been one continual interior martyrdom; all the powers and faculties of soul and body were sacrificed to God. After having suffered with Our Saviour here on earth, such a religious will be glorified with Him in heaven. Every step she made to visit the sick, every word of consolation uttered by her lips, every service rendered near the sick-bed, every wound she dressed and cured, every pain she soothed— all, all has been registered in the book of life by her guardian angel. And as God never allows Himself to be outstripped in generosity, but most liberally repays a hundred and a thousandfold whatever we do or suffer for Him, who can describe the reward which awaits such a religious! Her heavenly crown will be adorned with as many pearls and precious stones as there have been invalids whom for God's sake she has tended and prepared for a happy end. Her very body will be transfigured and glorified on the Last Day. Every sense, every member will receive its own reward:

those eyes which gazed so compassionately on loathsome wounds and ulcers will contemplate the splendor of the divine Majesty; those ears which many a night heard the groans and sighs of the dying will be ravished by the enchanting music of the celestial choirs; those lips constantly opened to speak words of instruction, encouragement, or consolation will now unite with the angels and saints in singing canticles of praise and thanksgiving to God for that sublime vocation in which they found their happiness and their eternal salvation ; those hands indefatigable in rendering the meanest services to the sick will shine with a splendor far surpassing all earthly beauty.

CHAPTER III.

The Service of the Sick a Difficult Vocation.

IT is by no means easy to comply perfectly with
the numerous demands made on an infirmarian;
this vocation imposing many arduous duties which
can only be faithfully performed by those who
possess the following requisite qualities and virtues :

I. QUALITIES REQUIRED IN A GOOD INFIRMARIAN:
FIRST, SOUND HEALTH OF BODY ; SECOND, QUIET
VIGILANCE ; THIRD, PERSEVERING COURAGE ;
FOURTH, PRUDENCE.

These qualities of course are partly the result
of natural disposition ; but in a Catholic infirmarian they must be ennobled, sanctified, and increased so that the manner of dealing with the
sick may become a true act of virtue.

1. It is very evident that an infirmarian must be
of a strong and *robust constitution*. It would be
impossible for a weakly or delicate person to bear
with the exigencies legitimately required of an
infirmarian; bad air, watching, and other heavy

duties would soon tell upon his health, nay, even upon his life.   In like manner the sick-nurse should not have about him anything which emits a strong odor and which might inspire the sick with disgust or repugnance. " The senses of an infirmarian," says Dr. Capellmann, "must be acute: he must be able to hear with ease even the faintest words of an enfeebled invalid; his eye must be clear in order to observe every change in the sick; his smell keen and sharp, so as to be himself the first to discern and expel foul air. This, as well as the sense of taste, he requires in order to examine and superintend the food and drink of the sick. A delicate sense of touch will also be of great use to enable him to discern the higher or lower degree of temperature in the invalid; it will enable him also to handle the sick man dexterously, so as not to cause him pain or discomfort."

2. In order to tend the sick successfully, great *vigilance* is needed. Above all things it is requisite that everything should be carefully avoided which in the smallest degree might be unpleasant or disagreeable to the invalid. Extreme cleanliness in their own persons is strongly recommended to infirmarians. In this regard the sick are often more susceptible than people in health; the least sign of uncleanliness, the slightest unpleasantness of smell, especially that of snuff or tobacco, is at once noticed and often suffices to tempt them to impatience and give them an aversion to their nurse.

This vigilance must also be exercised in studying the individual disposition and character of
the invalid, so as not to do or say anything which
might in any way offend him. For this end the
infirmarian must endeavor to learn, by assiduous
observation, whether the invalid is pleased to have
some one in attendance upon him, or whether he
prefers being left alone; whether such or such a
service should be offered to him, or whether it
should be rendered without his perceiving it;
whether he likes to be listened to, or whether he
prefers listening to others speaking. Generally
speaking, it may be taken as a rule that one must
play with children, chat with women, and speak
little with men. Indeed when tending the sick one
must imitate a devoted nurse, who understands not
only what the child says or means to say, but who
understands and divines its wants and wishes
from its very eyes, face, and movements. Thus,
also, when tending the sick it often happens that
from the mere demeanor of the invalid we can
know when he wishes to change his position or to
be raised in his bed, when he is thirsty, when the
air or temperature of the room does not agree with
him, etc.

This vigilance also involves a minute observation of the state of the sick man; for instance,
how he has slept, whether he changes color,
whether chilliness or perspiration has set in, what
effect food or medicine has wrought in him, and
such like things. By minute observation and experience we must also learn how to treat an invalid

differently in different cases; for example, whether to give him a drink in a spoon, or in a saucer, or in an invalid's cup, or whether we have simply to moisten his lips and thus to quench his thirst.

A love of order is also necessary to be able always to act with the requisite vigilance. Thus let it be an inviolable rule that everything has a fixed place and is returned to it as soon as it is no longer wanted. According to an old and very true proverb, order saves time and trouble. A place for everything and everything in its place. Moreover, it must be held as a principle that an object that has been used should never be put by without previously having been cleaned; thus it is preserved and can be used again. In fine, order and cleanliness are beneficial to the sick man, whereas the contrary is hurtful and displeasing to him.

Finally, quiet vigilance guards against precipitateness, which prevents us from doing a thing well. "Fair and softly goes far" is a golden rule which permits more and better work to be done.

3. To tend the sick with success, *persevering courage* is absolutely necessary. Without a considerable amount of patience and self-renunciation it is not possible to serve the sick properly according to the various changes of the malady, to comply with their various demands, and remain firm in difficult emergencies. Nothing should appall an infirmarian ; he should be ready to sacrifice even his life for the sick. He who is deficient in this spirit of self-sacrifice is like a soldier without

weapons; if he happens to meet with anything formidable, he will desert his post or do his duty badly. The infirmarian who wishes to act in a right spirit must not grow weary or show any impatience at the unreasonable complaints of the sick or their refractory conduct, nor be in any way disturbed by their continual petulance and fanciful humors; he must even be ready to bear patiently and quietly all kinds of injuries and reproaches. He must not show any disgust, nor shrink from rendering the lowliest services or handling what is most repulsive to his nature.

What heroic courage is required to dress wounds and ulcers, to bear nauseous smells, to assist at painful operations, to witness excruciating pain, to listen to heart-rending cries, which even the nearest relations are not able to endure !

Such resolute courage we admire in St. Jane Frances de Chantal, who was endowed by God with manly fortitude. One day while she still lived in the world they brought her a beggar covered with revolting ulcers, who had been found on the road. Madame de Chantal received this leper as a present from Heaven, cleansed his sores, dressed his wounds, and nursed him for four whole months, at the end of which time he died. With her own hands she laid him in the coffin, and when those present sought to prevent her from doing so, fearing she might take the infection, she made this beautiful answer: " I fear no other leprosy than that of sin."

4. As the service of the sick brings the infirma-

rian into a nearer contact with persons of all conditions, and as he has to be a helper and consoler
of the sick even in the most difficult circumstances, *prudence of conduct* is likewise an essential
requirement. Above all things infirmarians must
endeavor to acquire that exterior politeness of
manner which is found among persons of good
society, and which in their intercourse with the
poorer classes will gain them the respect which
is so desirable and often absolutely necessary for
their work. Their whole demeanor will bespeak
a modest dignity flowing from the consciousness
of the sublime nature of their duty and at the
same time, their own personal weakness. They will
moreover try to nurse the sick with ready devotedness and patience, and cheerfully bear with Christian prudence and charity their whims and fancies;
this condescension, however, must never induce
them to act contrary to the orders of the doctor.

Prudence requires that they should not speak unnecessarily with strangers about the nature of the
malady and its cause. As to the family concerns
of the invalids entrusted to their care, they should
not discuss them even with their fellow infirmarians, and much less with other people; they must
consider it as a sacred duty to observe an inviolable silence on such matters.

Prudence also forbids them to meddle with
family affairs, testamentary and other dispositions
regarding money, etc. The mere semblance of
such a proceeding should be scrupulously avoided.
Requests of this kind are to be discreetly declined

with the remark that such things are not in harmony with their calling, and that it is better to leave them to laymen who are more expert in such matters.

If the invalid or his friends desire the infirmarian to propose another doctor besides the one already in charge in order to consult him, he must observe most conscientious prudence and proceed with extreme caution and forbearance in this delicate matter.

In order not to give any cause of discontent either to the invalid or to his friends the infirmarian should carefully avoid leaving the house unnecessarily.

Familiar conversations and amusements with persons of the other sex, all mere worldly demonstrations of politeness and compliments must be carefully avoided. Infirmarians should also be cautious in giving or accepting small presents, such as pictures, etc., from the invalids.

They should never accompany invalids or convalescents to places of amusement where the presence of a religious person would be remarked or cause surprise. Nor should they ever allow themselves to be induced to go out driving or walking with persons of the other sex.

If the sick-nurse thinks the invalid is in danger of death, let him beware of announcing it suddenly and without due preparation; to many persons this would be an act of cruelty rather than a well-regulated charity which requires us to break this news, so awful to poor human nature, as gently as possible. In order not to frighten the invalid, but to familiarize him gradually with the thought of death, it is advisable to direct his thoughts to heaven, telling him how happy we should deem ourselves in being able to go there; that the time approaches when he will be called thither, and that it seems as though God were about to summon him speedily from this world, since the gravity of his illness leaves little or no hope of recovery. Remind him also that we cannot dwell forever on this earth; we must all die some day or other, and God wills that we should submit in this to His most holy decree. Then it would be well to exhort the sick man to consider these truths in his inmost heart.

II. VIRTUES TO BE PRACTISED WHILE TENDING THE SICK : FIRST, A LIVELY FAITH ; SECOND, CHARITY READY FOR ANY SACRIFICE ; THIRD, PRUDENT APOSTOLIC ZEAL ; FOURTH, INVINCIBLE PATIENCE.

1. *A Lively Faith.*—One who devotes himself to the care of the sick without being guided and animated by a spirit of faith will carry it on as a mere business, nay, even as a very irksome business, which easily irritates his temper and thus becomes hurtful both to the nurse and the sick person. But they who bear this yoke in the spirit of faith fulfil the arduous duties of their state willingly and joyfully through the motive of the love of God. Above all, the infirmarian finds power-

ful support and help in the words of our divine Saviour: " Whatsoever you do to the least of these My brethren, you do it unto Me." Faith shows him also in a vivid manner the dignity of the sick man entrusted to his care. He beholds in him a child of God created after God's own image and likeness, destined one day to inherit heaven, where he will praise and extol the Lord forever; he sees in his body, disfigured by suffering and illness, a living temple of the Holy Ghost and a member of Jesus Christ; he beholds in him, also, a soul—for whose redemption the Son of God came down from heaven, shed His precious blood, and died on the cross. In the light of faith, the infirmarian considers his office as one of the most excellent means of doing penance for his former sins, and of meriting a glorious reward in heaven for each loving service rendered to the sick. Moreover, by faith the nursing Brother and Sister are firmly convinced that, in the order of the superiors who allotted such or such an invalid to their care, the will of God is unmistakably made known, and that obedience will also provide them with the necessary graces to perform their office well for the good of the sick, and their own sanctification. Religious persons being called to imitate our divine Saviour in the most perfect manner possible, a good Brother or Sister of Charity will occasionally consider what Our Saviour would have done, how He would have conducted Himself, if He had met that poor, helpless invalid. With what heartfelt compassion would He have consoled him, with

what care would He have dressed his wounds
and done everything in His power to allay his pain
and prepare him for a happy passage into eternity!
Our Saviour no longer dwells on earth as in the
days of His earthly career; He Himself cannot
personally tend the sick person, but He has called
you, dear soul, consecrated to God, to render these
acts of charity to the invalid in His stead.

2. *Charity which is Ready for Sacrifice.*—It is
nothing extraordinary that a mother, a daughter,
or a wife should devote herself unreservedly to
the care of a sick child, a father, or a husband:
natural love inspires them with this spirit of sacrifice. It is also certain that sometimes, though
rarely, hired nurses are forgetful of their own
health : the hope of earning high wages urges
them to this. But to tend with the most devoted
care and affection an invalid who is a perfect
stranger, perhaps even badly disposed, to render
him the humblest services, and to do all this without any prospect of earthly reward or any signs of
gratitude, and that often at the risk of one's own
health—such love is to be found only in a soul
consecrated to the care of the sick through the
pure motive of the love of God. But such love
is truly *necessary* to the infirmarian to enable
him to accomplish his duty faithfully at all times;
to console and help the sick, sanctify himself in
his exalted but difficult calling, and store up a
large treasure of merits for heaven. It requires a
love undaunted by difficulties, a love devoted
without reserve to its work. This love manifests

itself especially in that compassion and delicacy which, with a watchful eye, see to all the wants of the patient, provide him with every alleviation both beneficial and agreeable, and carefully avoid everything that might annoy or displease him. This love is shown by a certain affability of manner, by gentle words, and by holy exhortations which like a soothing balm refresh the soul of the sufferer. It is further manifested by a constant readiness to render every possible service, despite the numerous demands, the ingratitude, nay, even the reproaches which are often to be met with from the sick. " Charity is patient, is kind; . . . it is not provoked to anger, thinketh no evil, . . . beareth all things, endureth all things " (1 Cor. xiii. 4–7).

One day the celebrated Franciscan, Bernardin de Feltre, gave a conference to the inmates of a large hospital. He took for his subject the maintenance and increase of mutual concord. Among other things he said: " Let each one read in *his own* little book so that he may learn what his duty is. In the book of the sick, it is true, we find everywhere the word ' Patience, patience, patience;' but in the book of the infirmarian a little word may likewise be found : ' Charity, charity, charity.' Let each one diligently read in *his own* little book and not seek to know what is written in that of the other. For if the sick man were always to be saying to the infirmarian: ' Where is your charity ? ' and the infirmarian to the poor sick man : ' Where is your patience ? '

they would be like children, each turning over
the leaves of his neighbor's book, without
studying the lesson in *his own,* and who
would have nothing to expect but punishment."
This maxim met with great approbation, and from
that time there were to be seen in each ward of
the hospital two tablets suspended on the walls;
the one bearing the thrice-repeated word " Charity "—the lesson for the infirmarians; the other
the thrice-repeated word " Patience "—the lesson
for the sick.

3. *Prudent Apostolic Zeal.*—While nursing the
sick it is of great importance that compassion for
the *bodily* sufferings of the sick should not make
us forget the care of *their souls;* in other words,
solicitude for the man must not make us forget
the care due to the Christian. It is true that the
spiritual care of the sick belongs principally to
the pastor. An unreasonable meddling in the interior affairs of the sick man is undoubtedly to be
blamed; nevertheless the care of the sick offers
many opportunities of preparing the way for the
pastor, especially as the priest cannot converse
with the invalid as often or as long as those who
are constantly with him.

The apostolic zeal of the infirmarian must first
of all show itself by preparing the sick person entrusted to his care for a pious reception of the
sacraments. Good Catholics do not, as a rule,
make much difficulty in this regard; but it is very
different with those who for years perhaps have
neglected their religious duties, have entirely

or partially lost their faith, or have burdened their consciences with so many sins of every kind that confidence in God's mercy appears quite impossible to them. In such cases the gentleness and kindness of the infirmarian can do much towards moving the invalid to a change of disposition and a return to God. To this end heartfelt compassion and kindly exhortations will do much more than reproachful moralizing. A well-known theologian says very aptly with respect to this matter : " An all-hoping mildness and a never-tiring longanimity gain their point and overcome even the most obdurate sinners; for they cannot resist the visible sorrow, the humble supplications, the gentle and discreet representations, the unceasing and hopeful efforts of love. Your love, compassion, and longanimity will touch and, in fine, gain their hearts. Even though your advances be repelled, though your loving words meet with contempt and harsh reply, be not indignant, nor grow angry; but go away only to return a little later. And then *come* and speak *again* with the same mildness, tranquillity, love, and hopefulness as before. If you be again turned away, come a third and a fourth time. For surely your mildness and long-suffering will at length find entrance and a willing ear." (Hirscher, Meditations, B. II., p. 265.) The human heart is so formed that it gives admittance only to love, and shrinks from harshness; it melts like wax in the genial rays of the sun, but hardens like clay in too great heat.

When the invalid has received the sacraments,

abundant opportunities present themselves to the infirmarian for exercising his apostolic zeal. The numerous duties of the pastor often prevent him from bestowing on each invalid the special and individual care he would wish in order to prepare him for a blessed end, to shield him against various temptations, and to point out to him the means of employing well the time of his illness and making it profitable for his soul. It is therefore the duty and privilege of the infirmarian who is constantly with the patient to seize every opportunity of performing this service of love, and to devote himself to so important a task. The manner in which this may best be done will be treated more at length in the second part of this book.

4. *Invincible Patience* is another virtue which must be practised in a high degree in the service of the sick.

In order that his illness may become a source of blessing and of merit, the invalid must be exhorted to patience and resignation to the will of God; and those who tend him must endeavor in every possible way to make the practice of this virtue easy to him. This may be best effected by their own patience and forbearance and by opposing a gentle and loving care to the discontent and impatience of the poor sufferer, remembering that, according to the designs of God, illness is intended to work out salvation and obtain merit not only for the sick, *but also for those who nurse him.* Moreover, let it not be forgotten that the care of the sick is in truth a *service.* Now, a service demands that one should be entirely at the disposal of him whom one has to serve. The service of the sick is often very hard and fatiguing; not infrequently it claims all one's time both day and night, leaving hardly a few spare minutes for repose; so that self-will has constantly to be renounced. How many sacrifices does the care of the sick involve ! You are tired and would be glad to rest a little, but duty requires that you should remain at your post; you would fain breathe a little fresh air, but it is impossible to leave the invalid; you must inhale bad and infected air; you would like to retire and pray, but you must work, hasten to and fro, toil and exert yourself; you are perfectly wearied and exhausted and can hardly stand erect, but you must be joyous, gay, affable, without betraying any interior struggle or repugnance. What demands are these on the patience of the infirmarian !

Many persons indeed know how to appreciate the loving care bestowed upon them; they shed tears of gratitude and emotion; but often, too, it happens that such services are repaid by rudeness and ingratitude, that the sick man, in his susceptibility or through some uncontrolled passion, gives way to murmurings and complaints, nay, perhaps lets himself be carried away so far as to make use of injurious and offensive language, and, as perchance it happens with persons diseased in mind, to commit acts of violence. In such cases it may easily be seen whether the infirmarian serves the sick from supernatural motives, by his not yielding to depression or ill humor, to anger or a secret spirit of revenge, but by his laying in an extra provision of love and patience. Instead of complaining of the invalid or treating him with indifference, let the infirmarian endeavor to find in his pitiable state an excuse for his failings, and, without betraying any aversion, let him try, as far as lies in his power, to please and cheer him up.

At times, however, a holy zeal and prudent energy have to take the place of patience. If a sick person were to go so far as to indulge in irreligious or unbecoming language, or were guilty of indecorous conduct, it would be but just, and a sacred duty, to reprove the guilty one with severity and manifest a holy indignation. But although vice be punished as it deserves, one must nevertheless continue to alleviate the misery of the delinquent. It was thus that our divine Saviour at first reproved the father of the lunatic boy: " O unbelieving and perverse generation ! how long shall I suffer you ? " (Matt. xvii. 16.) And yet He had compassion on him and healed the boy. But such a reprimand must be made only when it is absolutely necessary and the evil intention evident; for it sometimes happens that uneducated people allow themselves to pass remarks on religion without any bad intention; in such cases it is better not to answer with severity, but to instruct them charitably and lead them gently to a better frame of mind.

CHAPTER IV.

Tbe Service of tbe Sick a Dangerous Vocation.

It is very certain that the service of the sick is a high vocation, in which we can dispense many blessings and acquire treasures of virtue and merit; but on the other hand it cannot be denied that it is accompanied by a variety of dangers both for body and soul, and that, while serving others, we may do harm to ourselves.

I. DANGERS FOR THE SOUL.

1. In the first place there are dangers for the soul arising from *the immediate attendance* on the sick.

The sick-nurse has persons of every age and condition to tend; she has to render them a variety of services which easily lead the imagination to sinful thoughts; she is often obliged to remain both day and night for hours alone with the patient. How easy is it in such cases for weak virtue to suffer shipwreck if it is not firmly grounded in the fear of God, and if the soul is not penetrated with a lively faith in the presence of God ! One single

sinful look, a too natural attachment, or an un-
subdued passion is enough to plunge the soul into
the utmost danger. Doubtless God will not allow a person who in all sincerity tries, while serving the sick, to serve Him, to be tempted beyond
her strength. It is certain, I say, that He will not
allow a work of charity undertaken through obedience, to be the cause of that person's fall provided that nothing be wanting on her side, and
above all that she take every precaution and exercise a prudent reserve.

It would certainly betray a want of reserve as
well as of humility if, through vain presumption,
a person should boast that in the performance of
certain difficult services from which natural delicacy shrinks she experienced no pernicious impressions—that long habit had made her accustomed
and quite insensible to them. Such self-con-
fidence would be greatly displeasing to God, and
in many cases would draw down His chastisement,
which consists in humbling and defeating such
presumption. No, the sick should feel and know
that it is only through the love of God and in the
accomplishment of a holy duty that the sick-nurse
condescends to the various lowly services they require. On such occasions one who tends the sick
must show more than ever a holy gravity and carefully avoid everything that might stain the imagination or give rise to evil inclinations.

While nursing the sick one must conduct one's
self in such a manner as to deserve their gratitude for the charity and devotedness shown to

them, without, however, giving way to any kind of familiarity or too great tenderness, not only in one's actions, but also in one's endeavors to console or encourage them or entertain them with holy conversation. A friendly and cheerful manner is necessary to win the sick man and to alleviate his sufferings, but it must always be accompanied by a certain dignified gravity which inspires respect.

To the *Sisters of Charity* especially a quiet, serious affability is recommended, as well as reserve in speaking and the avoidance of all unbecoming familiarity in their dealings with the sick, the other infirmarians, the inmates of the house, the priest, and the medical attendants, so that they may fulfil the duties of their state without any danger to their own souls. Although they must give the physician an exact report as to the state of their patients, they should nevertheless keep within the bounds of the strictest reserve. They should never when possible converse with him except in the presence of others, nor be alone with him. This point is of the greatest importance, as it is when thrown in the company of doctors devoid of faith and morals that snares are often laid for the Sisters; special care must be taken when with young medical men who are strangers to them. Let them be on their guard, therefore, so that they may have no reason to regret inadvertencies which may prove fatal to their innocence. When good reasons demand it let them assist at surgical operations on female patients, but with regard to men let them assist only when such operations are made on the extremities of the body, that is, on the hands, arms, feet, and below the knee, or on the head and neck. The Sisters should not approach nearer to male patients any more than absolute necessity requires, nor stoop over them without need; they should not touch their hands, and should, in short, avoid everything contrary to the spirit of virginal modesty. In this respect they must not only think of the danger to which they expose themselves, but also of that into which they may plunge their patients. With regard to male patients who have been dismissed from their care they should under no pretext whatever continue any further intercourse with them, and still less should they go to visit them in their dwellings.

2. Besides the dangers which the nursing of the sick brings with it there are others which have their origin in human frailty, and often cause the sick-nurse while busy taking care of others to forget herself and *lose the true religious spirit.* Can a person who does not love himself truly love his neighbor ? Holy Writ asserts the contrary: " He that is evil to himself, to whom will he be good ? " (Ecclus. xiv. 5.) Nevertheless it often happens that religious who are devoted to the service of the sick give themselves up so unreservedly to exterior duties that they leave themselves no time to enter seriously into themselves; everything is done for others and nothing for their own souls. The melancholy consequences of such conduct are not difficult to see. How easy it is in such circumstances to nurture vanity,

selfishness, desire of human praise; in a word, a
love of the world ! How easily a distaste for God
and holy things creeps into the soul ! The soul
which was before all inflamed with the love of
God becomes tepid and lukewarm in His service,
the light of faith grows dimmer and dimmer, she
begins to act from purely natural motives, and
with this the spirit of sacrifice, so necessary for
the service of the sick, cannot long survive. She
continues to serve the sick, but only because it is
necessary in order to save appearances. Truly in
such persons the words of Our Saviour are verified,
for they are like those sepulchres which, although
outwardly beautiful, are " within full of death and
corruption " (Matt. xxiii. 27).

Our own sanctification is so essentially our first
duty that if we do not sanctify ourselves in the
service of our neighbor it would be better to relinquish this work of charity, and labor only at the
work of our own perfection. Thus it is that St.
Paul exhorts his disciple Timothy that in the administration of his pastoral duties he should first
and before all other things be mindful of his own
sanctification, and then devote himself to the
ministry and care of the flock entrusted to him.
In like manner the " Imitation of Christ " enjoins
us not to forget ourselves while working for
others; that is to say, that we should not neglect
our own perfection. To persons who, being occupied in works of charity, give themselves up too
much to exterior activity the words of Our
Saviour can very justly be applied: " What doth

it profit a man if he gain the whole world and suffer the loss of his own soul ? " Religious who are entrusted with the care of the sick are, on account of their constant bodily exertions, exposed to the danger of overfatiguing themselves, so that they are no longer able to perform their spiritual exercises in a suitable manner. The consequence is that when they go to meditation they can hardly refrain from falling asleep, and then they easily give way to the temptation of shortening or entirely omitting it. Vocal prayer, and in particular the Divine Office, meet with no better fate ; spiritual reading, if made at all, is done drowsily; the examination of conscience is made mechanically and without entering seriously into one's self; the Sacraments of Penance and of the Holy Eucharist are neglected without sufficient reason, or they are received with so much tepidity and indifference that the soul derives little or no benefit from them, relapsing continually into the same voluntary faults, and the heart insensibly grows more and more attached to the world and created things.

To guard against these dangers there is scarcely any better remedy than to make known one's state with childlike sincerity to one's superiors, and to the priest in the tribunal of penance. First of all, the religious should make known to her superiors the circumstances in which she lives, the difficulties she has to contend with, as well as the dangers resulting from them; let them be informed whether she is able to observe the rules, especially with regard to the exercises of prayer, spiritual readings, etc.; if prevented from doing so, she should ask for the requisite dispensation, in order always to preserve the spirit of obedience. When preparing for the Sacrament of Penance, let the religious seriously and carefully examine her conscience, remembering that God beholds the inmost recesses of the heart, and that even a slight attachment, if not suppressed in its very beginning, easily becomes a snare which may ruin a virtue of many years' standing. One should therefore never, under any pretext whatever, omit to tell the confessor, simply and candidly, everything that causes the soul uneasiness; otherwise the voice of conscience may by degrees be silenced and the soul brought to ruin. The chief aim of the enemy in such cases is to induce a person to conceal such dangers and temptations, that, being deprived of the help of a director, she may be left to her own blindness and frailty, and end in a fall.

II. DANGERS FOR THE BODY.

" Religious Communities devoting themselves to the service of the sick practise a kind of heroism," says Dr. Stoehr in his " Pastoral Medicine," " which deserves our admiration far more than all the legends of the heroes of ancient times, whose exploits in bygone days studied when we occupied the benches of a classroom, filled our youthful minds with enthusiasm. The more real the danger which is incurred by visiting the sick, the more joyfully the zeal of Catholic charity strives to give evidence that the Church now, as formerly, possesses numbers of combatants ready to die and to take their posts at all times in the field of battle. The history of each great epidemic exhibits martyrs of Christian charity to whom the palm is no less due than to those who sealed their faith with their blood. The hospital as well as the arena has its saints."

Notwithstanding all this we must not be unmindful of the dangers to which our life, or at least our health, is exposed while serving the sick, since no man is the absolute master of his life nor of the bodily strength given to him by God. A religious entrusted with nursing the sick has, it is true, entirely devoted him or her self to this service and must, if necessity requires it, be ready to sacrifice even his or her life in the accomplishment of this work of love. But, as everybody is obliged to take a reasonable amount of care for the preservation of health, this must be doubly applicable to religious, who no longer belong to themselves, but to the Community of which they are members. The dangers for the body in connection with the nursing of the sick may be reduced to three kinds.

They arise, first, from *too great fear ;* secondly, from *excessive exertion ;* thirdly, from a *neglect of precaution.*

1. Even in ordinary cases an undaunted courage is necessary in order to nurse the sick with success;

but it often happens that people who do not generally recoil from the care of the sick lose all their equanimity when required to attend those who are attacked by a contagious malady. Experience teaches that no one is in greater danger of taking infection than those who in such cases allow themselves to be overcome by excessive fear, the nervous system being thereby strongly affected and the body rendered more susceptible for imbibing the morbid matter. Even the most malignant contagious illnesses, such as the plague and the like, lose in part their dangerous character when they are encountered without fear. When in the seventeenth century the plague was raging at Marseilles, it vanished almost entirely as soon as a physician publicly declared that the evil was not contagious and attacked only the timid. In the same way the above-named Dr. Stoehr says: " This cheerful, God-confiding courage which, in its desire of helping, consoling, and saving, has not the time even to think of the possibility of infection; this childlike, unsuspecting courage, I say, which, following as it were the dictates of instinct, goes to meet the danger, is a better preservative against the transmission of an epidemic than the whole collection of disinfecting remedies of which modern science boasts." Therefore when going to the sick man make use of due precautions, but put aside all timidity and be not apprehensive of danger. And why, I ask, should you fear ? Those who through love of God, through genuine supernatural love of their neighbor, serve the sick.

are they not sheltered by a special protection of God ? Thus it rarely happens that infirmarians are attacked by dangerous maladies. And should they fall victims to them, they die martyrs of charity; and what death could be more glorious, more enviable ?

2. Young religious, especially in the beginning of their active lives, are exposed to the danger of not taking care of their health and bodily strength, and thus soon succumb to *over-exertion*. They take so much to heart the misery which they have every day before their eyes that, cost what it may, they are resolved to help and relieve the sufferers. So noble and generous a disposition is undoubtedly very beautiful and praiseworthy; but, just as God does not give us the means of helping all the poor in their necessities, so also in the service of the sick we must remain satisfied with rendering that amount of assistance that God has placed at our disposal. Unless for some very important reason, the infirmarian should never remain more than three or four weeks with the same invalid; at the end of that term he should allow himself to be relieved by others. An author experienced in the service of the sick gives the following noteworthy counsels: Let it be borne in mind that four hours of sleep spent in a good bed at night and out of the sick-room are of far greater value than eight hours' rest taken during the day. Moreover, for the sick man himself it is better to watch near him a day and a night without interruption than two nights with a day's rest between.

Finally, if three nights have been spent in watching, one whole night's rest at least should be taken, as well as a short time set apart each day for the same purpose.

3. Although the infirmarian in the service of the sick, which is so pleasing to God, may justly promise himself the special protection of Providence and need not fear too much for his own health, nevertheless Christian prudence demands that he should not expose himself unnecessarily to dangers by neglecting such *precautions* as physicians and long experience recommend. The principal safeguards may be briefly mentioned here:

Dr. Stoehr in his "Pastoral Medicine" advises us not to visit the sick when suffering ourselves from any indisposition. "A body which is already indisposed by having inhaled some morbid essence is peculiarly liable to imbibe contagious matter and, generally speaking, evinces but little power of resisting physical as well as moral disease."

When possible avoid going into the sick-room while yet fasting.

For the sick man as well as for his nurses a frequent renewal of pure air is absolutely necessary; but be on your guard not to expose the invalid to cold or draughts.

When speaking with a sick person, do not stand or sit face to face with him; on the contrary, let his head be in the same direction as yours, so that his breath may not come into immediate contact with your own.

When making the bed or changing the linen be careful not to inhale the perspiration.

If possible do not take your meals in the sick-room. Extraordinary exertions require very solid diet.

After having visited a suspicious invalid be sure to air your clothes by a turn in the open air, and inhale the pure air into your lungs by repeatedly drawing a long, deep breath. If possible try not to breathe through the mouth, but through the nose. The latter is as good as a filter with regard to the countless little atoms which fill the atmosphere. Strict observance of this rule proves in many cases a powerful safeguard against infection, since the germ of many an infectious disorder finds its way into the body by means of the breath.

During epidemics care should be taken not to enter the sick-room while in a state of heat or perspiration. It is further advisable to chew the root of the angelica plant, or from six to ten juniper-berries a day ; to expectorate the saliva which is formed in the mouth while with the invalid; and finally, after the visit, to rinse the mouth with vinegar and water, and wash the hands and face.

Many contagious diseases, such as those of a scabious nature, hydrophobia, etc., are propagated only through the touch; you are therefore quite safe from infection as long as you do not touch in a direct manner either the invalid or the things infected by him. In such cases even the atmosphere, as well as everything that has been in the neighborhood of the sick man, should be carefully avoided; hence fumigations, renewal of the air, and other such means of disinfection should be resorted to.

CHAPTER IV. (CONTINUED.)

Striking Examples for Infirmarians.

1. The great leper hospital of Cæsarea, founded
about the year 372 by *St. Basil*, archbishop of that
city, filled the East with the fame of his charity.
His love for the sick was so great that he used
to embrace them as brothers, and this not through
a motive of vanity, which was quite foreign to
him, but in order to lessen the repugnance felt by
his companions to touch and to assist these unfortunate creatures. He founded this establishment
on so grand a scale that, in addition to the wards
for the sick, there was ample accommodation for
doctors, guards, attendants, and porters, and even
all the more useful and necessary artisans had
their dwellings and workshops there. The Emperor Valens, who was at first prejudiced against
the saint, later on became so prepossessed in his
favor that he made over to the hospital the choicest tracts of land which he owned in the neighborhood.

2. At Hohenberg in Alsatia there lived at the

beginning of the eighth century the holy abbess *Odilia.* One day she found at the gate of the monastery a leper so repulsive that no one durst approach him. The saint, however, took him in her arms, gave him some food with her own hands, and nursed him, beseeching God with tears to grant him either the cure of his malady or patience to bear his sufferings, whereupon the sick man was immediately restored to health.

3. The saintly *Countess Sybilla,* daughter of Fulk, King of Jerusalem, was in the year 1134 married to Theodoric, Count of Flanders. On Theodoric's third expedition to Jerusalem he took his wife with him, and while her husband joined the crusaders in fighting against the infidels, she retired to the convent of St. Lazarus, where with wonderful patience and self-denial she tended the poor invalids. She washed and dressed the wounds of the lepers and others with her own hands, and when her nature revolted she took, by way of self-chastisement, into her mouth some of the water she had used, and as she swallowed it said to herself: " You are to serve God in their person, and this is to be your employment forever, even though you should break down under the burden." When after a few years her husband returned to Flanders, she besought him earnestly to allow her to offer herself in sacrifice to God and spend the remainder of her life in the convent, serving the sick; which request, at the intercession of her royal brother and other friends, was at length granted to her.

4. *Alquirinus*, a Cistercian monk, applied himself with such fervor to the care of the sick that he touched their wounds as though he were handling the most precious pearls and sweet-smelling balsam. And God rewarded the fraternal charity of this holy religious not merely by interior consolations, and by converting the offensive smell of the wounds into a celestial odor, but at the end of his life He gave him also to understand how pleasing this beautiful work of charity had been to Him. When he lay on his death-bed, Alquirinus was filled with a holy calm and joy, and, in spite of the severity of his illness, he appeared to suffer nothing. The abbot, not a little surprised, ordered him to reveal the cause of his joyfulness. Upon which he replied: " Be it known to you, Father, that Christ has appeared to me, and, assuring me of my everlasting bliss, He invited me to kiss His most holy wounds, which I have so often and so lovingly tended in the person of His servants. Why, then, should I not rejoice now, since this night, while my brethren are in choir, my soul will rise to the enjoyment of everlasting felicity ? " And so indeed it happened.

5. The tremendous inundations and the scarcity which at the beginning of the thirteenth century afflicted all Silesia were followed by a great famine and a variety of diseases. *St. Hedwig* did her best to render assistance to the unfortunate people, but more especially to the lepers. In a house near the town of Neumarkt she placed several leprous

women who would otherwise have wandered about in the fields and desert places and come to a miserable end. Several times each week she used to send them money, food, clothes, and other things, and for Christ's sake she considered and treated them in all respects as her beloved daughters. Although frequently ill herself and of a delicate constitution, she nevertheless overcame her natural repugnance, knelt down by the sick, washed and cleansed their ulcers, and beholding in them the wounds of her Saviour, she would press her lips to them in order to suck the foul matter from the sores.

6. *St. Francis of Assisi* before entering the religious life was one day riding through the plain of Assisi, when to his horror he beheld a loathsome leper approaching him. He at once sprang from his horse and hurried to meet the unfortunate man, who was holding out his hand for an alms. Francis gave him some money and embraced him. But on remounting his horse, the leper was no longer anywhere to be seen. Then he felt within his heart a deep interior joy, and he rode along his way singing the praises of God. He, who till then had had so intense a horror of lepers that he was ready to flee away at the mere sight of one, was now so filled with the love of our divine Saviour that everywhere he went in search of those unfortunate creatures and rendered them the lowliest services. He washed their feet, cleansed their ulcers from the foul matter, and dressed and kissed their sores with the most

touching fervor. His holy manner of life being already noised abroad, he one day met a poor leper from the county of Spoleto whose jaw-bone and mouth were most horribly disfigured. The unfortunate man, who had had recourse to all kinds of remedies, was just returning from a pilgrimage to Rome. When he met the saint, he cast himself down in his misery to kiss his feet. Francis, whose humility could not suffer this, raised him up from the ground and, clasping him in his arms, kissed the ghastly wounds in his face, whereupon the sick man completely regained his health.

7. *St. Elizabeth of Hungary*, Landgravine of Thuringia, had a singular predilection for lepers. One Holy Thursday she caused all the lepers of the neighborhood to be assembled. She then washed their hands and feet, and on her knees devoutly kissed their sores and ulcers. One day a leper presented himself who suffered also from a malady in his head. The young landgravine had him laid in the garden, and did what very probably the most wretched beggar woman would not have done even for a large reward. She laid his head on her lap, and cutting off his hair, which was clotted with matter, she washed and dressed his head. While she was thus engaged, her maids of honor came to meet her, and instead of being ashamed or disconcerted, Elizabeth laughed heartily: true Christian virtue being always cheerful and performing any good work as if it were a matter of course. Another time, in the

absence of the landgrave, Elizabeth availed herself of the opportunity to devote all her time and
energy to the care of the sick poor. Her mother-
in-law, Sophia, was greatly displeased at this; for
in the eyes of the world nothing appears more ab-
surd and intolerable than to see a noble princess
exercising a maternal care towards the poorest and
most wretched creatures and tending them as
though they were her own children ! One day she
happened to meet a leper small of stature and at
the same time so disfigured and repulsive in his
appearance that no one would have anything to
do with him. Now this was for Elizabeth a happy
meeting. She took him with her, bathed and
anointed his sores, and laid him in her own bed.
While she was thus tending the poor man her
husband arrived. Immediately the old landgravine,
his mother, ran to meet him, uttering loud complaints against Elizabeth. " Only come and see,"
she said, " what wonders your Elizabeth is doing";
and taking him by the hand she led him into his
bedroom, adding: " Just see, dear son, your wife
lays lepers in your bed without allowing any one
to prevent her; it seems as if she wanted to make
a leper also of you." Full of indignation, the
landgrave drew back the bed-curtain, and whom
should he behold but Jesus Christ crucified !
Elizabeth stood behind her husband, considering
in her own mind how she could appease his anger;
but he with a smiling countenance turned to her
and said: " Elizabeth, my dear sister, you may
often put such guests into my bed; I shall be very

grateful for it. Let no one hinder the performance of your acts of charity."

8. Besides the numerous favors which *St. Lewis*
bestowed upon the leper hospitals, he made it a
pious custom to visit these establishments on the
ember-days, and offered the most touching proofs
of fraternal charity to those " poor children of
God " who were stricken with leprosy. He fed
them with his own hands, and kissed their festering hands and feet.

9. The holy abbess *St. Mechtildis* used to tend
her sick sisters with true maternal care. However much she might be occupied, she went to
visit them daily; with her own hands she served
and procured them every possible relief. When
she was advanced in years and no longer able to
walk, and she herself carried to the poor sufferers,
so highly did she esteem the sick, and so great
was her zeal to serve the afflicted members of
Christ.

10. *St. Catharine of Sienna,* having heard of a
very poor woman named Cecha who was attacked
by a frightful leprosy and was utterly destitute,
hastened to offer her help and support to the poor
creature, and attended her with the devoted care
of a most loving child. She fed her, washed,
cleansed, and dressed her wounds day after day,
and bore the ghastly sight and awful stench of the
loathsome wounds of the poor sick woman with so
much cheerfulness that one would have imagined
she was the most amiable of invalids. But the
Lord, wishing to try the patience of His spouse,

as He tried holy Job of old, allowed the spirit of darkness to assail Cecha with the most violent temptations. Covered with leprosy in her body, she appeared to be still more leprous in her soul. She made no other return to the devoted charity of the saint than continual anger, murmuring, sarcasm, insults, and shameful calumny. One day Catharine went a few minutes later than usual to visit her, and was received with a volley of abuse. Her ill humor increased with her malady, but so did Catharine's patience and unwearying care. But the Lord was pleased to test the virtue of His spouse still further, and permitted Catharine's hands to be attacked with leprosy. And now every one blamed the saint for having brought upon herself so terrible a malady, and fled from her for fear of contagion. But all these tribulations were unable to disturb her peace of mind; and she joyfully acquiesced in the divine will, receiving the leprosy and all the murmurings and reproaches that resulted from it from the hand of God, feeling that she was thereby rendering herself more like to her heavenly Spouse. After she had patiently and cheerfully borne this trial for some time, the Lord was pleased to release His pious servant both from the cruel malady with which she was afflicted and from the arduous duty which her charity had undertaken. Cecha's end was approaching, and Catharine redoubled her zeal for the salvation of her soul. After the poor woman had breathed her last, Catharine completed her work of love by preparing the horribly disfigured and repulsive corpse of Cecha for burial. She washed it with her own hands, clothed it in clean linen, and laid it out decently upon the bier. This work of charity being done, she looked down at her own hands, and lo, they were as free from disease as the hands of a new-born babe ! And in token of the divine approbation, the places on her hands which had been attacked by the leprosy were particularly clean and bright, as if a soft light issued from them.

11. In the year 1400 a terrible plague broke out in Italy. *St. Bernardine of Sienna* was then in his twentieth year. In Florence alone about eight hundred persons died daily; and it was not long before the black death made its appearance also at Sienna. At St. Mary's Hospital in that town from twelve to sixteen persons were carried off each day, and this state of things continued for months. Added to this, the attendants entrusted with the care of the sick were attacked with the same malady, and nearly all fell victims to the plague, as well as nine priests, twenty-two Brothers of Charity, five clerics, several doctors, thirty-six boys who dwelt in the hospital, besides sixty servants and many brave and virtuous citizens who had nobly offered their services. In a word, the hospital had become a place of horror, an atmosphere of pestilence, where nothing was to be seen on all sides but the dead and the dying. No one would venture to be engaged as an infirmarian, not even for a large sum of money, and the invalids cried in vain for help and mercy. It was

then that Bernardine felt within himself the desire
to hasten to the assistance of the poor, abandoned,
pest-stricken inmates of the hospital. Fearless of
death, he went to the director of the hospital and
asked, for the love of Jesus and Mary and for the
sake of a heavenly reward, to be permitted to serve
the poor inmates. His offer being thankfully accepted, Bernardine set to work with a resolute
heart, full of joy and zeal, and labored indefatigably for the good of his fellow-creatures. In order
to purify the air, great fires were lit in the court-
yard, and the house was thoroughly fumigated.
Bernardine was everywhere and always the first to
set a good example. Nothing abated his fervor,
neither the offensive odor, the filth and dirt, nor
fatigue, nor the fear of death. With his own
hands he removed the pus from the plague-boils,
dressed and buried the dead, acting towards all,
not as a superior, but as a father and a loving
brother. In the person of each one entrusted to
his care he revered and served Jesus Christ Himself. But what gave a peculiar stamp of nobleness
to all he did, and increased his merit, was the fact
that he had to suffer persecution on account of
his heroic charity. His noble relatives were displeased at his devoting himself so unreservedly to
the service of the sick, and were not satisfied with
using every kind of remonstrance to dissuade him
from pursuing his holy purpose, but indulged in
bitter complaints, calling him a madman for thus
needlessly exposing his life. But these proceed-
ings were only an incentive for Bernardine to

continue with greater ardor to serve the sick, for he had now a double reward in view: one for his active charity, the other for the persecution he was enduring.

12. *St. Roch*, after having distributed his patrimony among the poor, secretly left his home to go to Rome as a pilgrim and a beggar. On his way he came to Aquapendente in Tuscany, where a most dangerous and pestilential malady was then raging. Without delay he offered himself to render the lowliest services to the sick. He did the same at Rome, where with heroic charity he attended the pest-stricken for about three years. Thence he returned to the places where he had previously been, and everywhere he devoted himself to serving the most forlorn of the sick. At Piacenza, where likewise a kind of contagion had broken out, he again offered himself to nurse the sick in the hospital.

13. One day *St. John of God* found a dying man lying in the street. He gently lifted him up on his shoulders, and carrying him to his hospital, laid him on a good bed and washed his feet. While he was stooping down devoutly to kiss his feet, he perceived an uncommon brightness, and on raising his eyes he recognized Jesus Christ, who said to him: " John, charity which is exercised towards the poor is done to Me. I stretch out My hand to receive the alms that are given; I am clothed with the garments which are bestowed on the indigent; and it is My feet you wash each time you render this loving service to a poor person." This

vision filled John's heart with heavenly joy, and inspired him with a great desire to give himself up entirely to the service of the poor. There were a number of patients in his hospital, of every age and sex, afflicted with all kinds of disorders. No one was refused admittance, however malignant and infectious his malady might be. He also received all the foundlings, lunatics, and idiots that were sent to him. As he was much occupied, it was often late at night when he returned to the hospital. But, however tired he might be, he did not go to rest before he had visited each one of his patients, inquired if anything was required by them, and shown them the most tender sympathy. On one great festival day a fire broke out in the hospital and spread with such rapidity and violence that it caught the upper stories, where the sick lay exposed to the utmost danger. The whole town ran to witness the catastrophe, but none durst attempt to save the unfortunate people from death. The servant of God alone pierced the crowd, and, seeing the danger which threatened his poor sick people, forced his way through smoke and fire and carried out all the invalids, one after the other. Then he hurried back to save the beds and furniture, throwing them out of the windows with wonderful activity, and penetrated even under the roof, where the fire enveloped him on all sides, until he disappeared from the wondering gaze of the multitude. For half an hour he remained wrapped in the flames; then he reappeared unscorched. This event was generally looked upon as a miracle, and the Church itself perpetuates the memory of St. John's heroic deed, alluding to it in the office of his feast, where it is said that the love of God which filled his heart caused him to walk through the flames without suffering any harm.

14. *St. Camillus* was born in the kingdom of Naples and descended from the noble family of the Lelli. Like his father, he chose to be enrolled in the army from his early youth. In his profession he was unfortunately for some time engaged in the ways of sin. But at the age of twenty-five, on the feast of the Purification of our blessed Lady, the grace of God touched him so powerfully that he completely turned to God, and, renouncing the world, devoted himself entirely to the service of the sick at Rome, where, in the hospital for incurables, he engaged himself as infirmarian. In this position he made himself so remarkable for his zeal and shining virtues that he was raised to the dignity of a warden. When any one of the sick was nearing his end, he ceased not his pious exhortations until he had fittingly prepared him for death by a worthy reception of the last sacraments. Being ordained priest, his zeal in the care of the sick and dying went on increasing and was the cause of his instituting the Order called "the Regular Clerics for the Service of the Sick," whose members by a special vow obligate themselves to serve the plague-stricken. When he was at Nola and at Rome, where a formidable plague was raging, he

used to carry the sick on his shoulders into the hospital, in spite of his weak health and a festering ulcer on his foot from which he continually suffered; and St. Philip Neri saw angels descending from heaven to whisper into his ear words of consolation for the sick and dying. In spite of his great weakness, which hardly allowed him to walk, he dragged himself to the beds of the sick to console them, and to sinners to reconcile them with God. Hospitals, battle-fields, lazarettos, and private houses were alternately the theatre of his heroic charity. After having distinctly predicted the hour of his death, he expired (1614) at the moment when the attending priest was reciting the prayer of the Church for the dying: " May Jesus Christ appear to thee with a mild and cheerful countenance, and appoint thee a place among those who are to stand before Him forever."

Pope Leo XIII. declared him patron of the sick and hospitals, and ordained that henceforward he should be expressly invoked in the Litany of the Dying.

15. It was in the spirit of humility and mortification that *St. Francis Borgia,* like a charitable Samaritan, devoted himself to the care and consolation of the sick. Knowing well from personal experience what illness was, he was full of compassion for the suffering patients, and with his own hands he gave them all possible relief. In the hospital at Madrid he not only devoted himself to preaching, hearing confessions, and preparing the sick for a good death, but he also used every

means in his power to afford them relief in their
pains. He washed their hands and feet with all
the diligence and attention of a most loving
mother towards her children, and after having
cleansed them well with water and pared the nails
he poured a fragrant lotion over them, and kissing them he honored in them the blessed hands
and feet of his divine Master. He then cut the
hair of those who needed it, and made their beds.
Special mention is made of a poor sick woman
whose hair he cut with extreme care and patience,
and delivered her at the same time from the vermin which had caused her as much suffering as her
disease. Moreover, he gave food to the sick,
making use of the most loving and ingenious con-
trivances in order to overcome their natural repugnance for nourishment. This being done, he
went to the kitchen to serve as a scullion, and remained there until all the utensils that had been
used were cleansed.   Then he returned to the
hospital, and, going from bed to bed, attended to
each poor invalid and washed and cleansed to the
best of his power whatever had been used by them.

16. Besides several other charitable institutions,
St. Charles Borromeo also founded various hospitals. Although archbishop and cardinal, he nevertheless went in person to visit and console the
sick, gave them the sacraments, and assisted the
dying. It was especially during the plague which
in the year 1566 raged for several months at Milan
that the holy archbishop displayed this loving solicitude for the sick. Being advised and urged,

in order to preserve his life, to quit the city until the cessation of the plague, he would not consent, answering only to such importunities: " I am the shepherd, and a good shepherd giveth his life for his sheep." Resolved to give his life for his flock, he stayed in the city, and not only shared the danger with them, but also took care that those attacked by the pestilence should be tended in the best possible manner with regard to body and soul. He sent priests into all the streets of the city, that they might be ready to administer the sacraments to the sick, so that none might die without the last consolations of the Church. He himself went in preference into the houses of the poorer class, heard their confessions, gave them the last sacraments, and provided for their bodily necessities. At that time many a family was in the utmost need, for victuals were no longer brought into the city, and the stores grew daily less. Even in this distress the holy archbishop came to the relief of the unfortunate inhabitants. He had all his own provisions of corn and other victuals distributed among the needy; he sold his silver-plate and furniture, and gave away in alms the money he thereby obtained. He did not even spare his clothes nor the fine carpets in his palace. In the end his own bed went to the hospital, while he made use of a hard board for his night's rest.

17. *St. Peter Claver, S.J.*, with heroic charity took in hand the interests of the poor negro slaves. One day he was called to one of them, who, on

account of the offensive nature of his ulcers, had
been removed to the farthest corner of the house.
At the first sight of this unfortunate creature, the
servant of God, being overpowered with repugnance, shrank back.   But, as though ashamed of
this involuntary revolt of nature, he retired awhile,
and, thinking himself alone and unobserved,
cast himself on his knees, and after a short and
fervent prayer gave himself a severe discipline.
Then returning to the sick man, he knelt down
and kissed all his wounds; he then heard his confession, and stayed with him several hours more
in order to nurse and console him.   The master of
the slave and several other gentlemen, who had
secretly watched Father Claver, were astonished
beyond measure at such heroism; they had seen
a saint grow weak for a moment, but only to redouble the fervor of his charity.   Prayer imparts
courage and strength even to the weak.

18. *St. Vincent of Paul* when parish priest at
Chatillon (1617) founded an "Association of
Christian Charity," composed of ladies who devoted themselves to the bodily and spiritual care
of the sick poor.   Later on, during his missions,
he often met with souls who, disinclined for the
things of this world, would fain have consecrated
their lives to the service of God, but felt no inward call to enter a convent.   He consulted the
venerable servant of God Louise de Marillac,
Madame Le Gras, on the subject, and they mutu-
ally determined (1632) to unite such persons in a
kind of society, the members of which, like the

above-mentioned Association, should devote themselves to the care of the sick. This was the origin
of the Congregation of the " Sisters of St. Vincent
of Paul," who have spread over all the countries
of the world and now number about twenty-seven
thousand. St. Vincent enjoined them to consider themselves merely the servants of Christ,
chosen to tend their divine Redeemer in the person of the poor and the sick. As such they should
be indefatigable in the pursuit of perfection, do
all their works in the spirit of humility and Christian simplicity, through love of God, in union
with the actions of Our Saviour during His mortal
life, and without any regard for the praise or ap-
plause of men. In the year 1658 he sent four
Sisters to Calais, where hundreds of soldiers were
dying of their wounds or of contagious maladies;
two Sisters succumbed to the fatigue, but twenty
others offered themselves to replace them. " See
the providence and goodness of God," wrote the
saint, " who at this time had made choice of such
a Community. Is it not a touching thing and
very meritorious before God to see these virgins
go with so much courage and devotedness among
the soldiers to assist them in their wants and to
promote the salvation of their souls; to see them
expose themselves to suffering, to dangerous maladies, and even to death ? " The numberless institutions for the relief of suffering humanity,
especially the poor and sick, which had been
founded by St. Vincent obtained for him an immortal fame; and Pope Leo XIII. (1885) declared

him " Patron of all the Works and Associations of Christian Charity."

19. The charity of *St. Francis Regis* seemed to redouble whenever he saw poverty go hand in hand with illness. It was because he considered himself deputed by God to be the nurse of all the poor and oppressed, the sick and needy; wherefore also there was no kind of charitable work which he did not undertake. How well the sick poor appreciated this devoted generosity may be inferred from their conviction that they would find relief if they could but obtain a sight of their good father, whom they looked upon as an angel sent to them by God. Although he could not free them entirely from their pains, nevertheless he was able in some degree at least to alleviate them. There was no service of charity that he did not readily perform for them. He might be seen carrying to them bedding, straw, mattresses, clothes, and various articles of furniture, and he did this with as much joy as if it were indeed the adorable person of Jesus Christ, his divine Master, that he was serving. In a miserable hut on the outskirts of the town of Le Puy lay a poor man dangerously ill. He was so covered with ulcers and vermin that he inspired not only abhorrence but even terror; and if any one ventured to approach to render him any service, he was repulsed by the insupportable stench. The report of his most distressing situation reached at length the ears of our saint, who at once hastened to the unfortunate man, and at the sight of such untold misery burst out weep-

ing. But he did not confine himself to such
mere demonstrations of sympathy: he dressed his
wounds, washed with his own hands his clothes
and bedding, and provided him with a decent bed.
Day by day he returned to dress his wounds and
to strengthen him with food and drink. In token
of his gratitude the poor man one day called the
servant of God his father and redeemer. Deeply
moved, the saint fell on his neck and, pressing
him to his heart, exclaimed : " Ah ! my dear
friend, it is for me to thank you; for I derive
greater benefit from these small services than you
do. The little I do for you is nothing in com-
parison with what I should wish to do. One
thing only I ask of you: forgive me for having
come so late to see you."

20. The servant of God, *Philip Teningen, S.J.*
(d. 1704), made himself remarkable by his devoted love for the sick. Whether called or not,
he went to see them and offered them help whenever he could. But in the case of those who were
dangerously ill or dying, he left at once every
other occupation and went to their bedsides.
It frequently happened that, on returning wearied
from a mission or leaving the confessional
at noon fasting, he was told that some one seriously ill desired to see him. Then, without rest
or food, he would immediately set out, and remain with the patient as long as he could be of
any use to him.

In the hospital at Ellwangen there was a poor
man who was suffering from a terrible ulcer,

which was constantly festering and causing him violent pain. On account of the offensive smell no one would nurse the poor invalid. This excited the compassion of the servant of God. Embracing the unfortunate man, he consoled him, threw himself at his feet, kissed the ulcer, and sucked out the matter. This heroic act he repeated four times.

To prevent his sick from dying without the sacraments, the holy priest performed daily a certain devotion in honor of St. Barbara, and through her intercession obtained what he prayed. for. There is not a single case on record of a person under his spiritual direction departing this life without the last sacraments. Let us mention only one among the many remarkable incidents of this kind.

A woman having been ill for some time, and feeling that her end was near, asked her husband to send for Father Teningen to give her the sacraments. The surly man declared this to be a mere whim and exaggeration, and absolutely refused to comply with her request. Not long after, her agony in very truth commenced. Of course Father Teningen was now sent for, but on his arrival the sick woman was already in her agony. Full of confidence, Father Teningen began by invoking St. Barbara, whereupon the invalid recovered consciousness and sufficient strength to enable her to make a full confession of her sins and receive the last sacraments, shortly after which she died.

21. Even when still in the world *St. Alphonsus Maria di Liguori* used to visit the sick in the hospitals, to console and render them the most abject services. This love of the sick he continued to practise later on when a bishop, and persevered in it to a great age. When he heard of poor people confined to their beds by illness, the loving pastor provided them with food and necessaries ; nay, sometimes he would take them preserves and other delicacies. Every evening he rose from his work to go and see the sick, of whatever condition they might be, and prepare the dying for a good death. Of this a priest who had been an eye-witness gives the following account: " I could not sufficiently admire his great love for the sick. Although seventy-seven years old, infirm and paralyzed, he nevertheless used to go about in the town of Arienzo to visit the sick. The sight of an old man whose head was so bent that his chin almost rested on his chest, trembling in all his limbs, who was himself every day visited by two physicians, and yet in this state went to visit the poorest people in their humble dwellings—this sight, I say, filled me with admiration. I always looked upon it as an heroic act of virtue, and could not behold it without tears rising to my eyes."

22. *Bishop Wittmann* when still provost of the cathedral (1813) of Ratisbon took pleasure in performing the functions of chaplain to the military hospital. He himself owned that in the months of October and November he exposed his life to imminent danger in the hospital. He spent whole

days in the lazaretto, hearing confessions and administering the sacraments to the sick and dying. At the beginning of December he was taken ill with typhus fever, which did not abate until February, 1814, when there appeared no hope of recovery. Yet, though himself little concerned about his recovery, God preserved his life and suddenly restored him to health, as he himself declares in his diary.

This holy priest, while giving himself up to the care of the sick, always did it in a spirit of real servitude, as he used to say, and he extended his activity in the hospitals to the work of distributing and carrying fuel to and fro like a servant. It is generally believed that when the Jesuits' house was on fire he carried out and saved from the flames the sick and especially the invalid soldiers. He also assisted the wounded in the streets amidst a shower of bullets, and gave many similar proofs of his courage and apostolic zeal. He provided the necessary linen, and when at times a great scarcity was felt in the hospital he went about collecting from house to house, and never left the hospitals of the sick without distributing some gifts. If a sick man asked him for a rosary, he always gave it ; if for a book of devotion, he seldom refused. In short, he applied himself to the service of the sick with the same assiduity as to any other of his duties, so that it might have been supposed he had only to attend to this business and to no other.

His zeal for the sick in hospitals was equalled

by that for the sick in private houses, especially
for such as were poor and destitute, of whom
there were a great many at Ratisbon. Great was
his affliction when he found no means of assisting
them, and he ceased not to call on God to enable
him to find some charitable souls who would provide for the abandoned; he applied to kind-hearted
people and prevailed upon them to take charge of
the poor forsaken invalids during the winter. Yet
he did not exhort by words only, but also by example. He once had in the poorhouse a very
aged and infirm widow, who in her protracted
illness constantly needed attendance. To practise
self-denial, mortification, and humility, Wittmann
took the care of this person almost entirely upon
himself. He went every day at a fixed hour, and
acquitted himself of every service, however repulsive it might be. He gave her food and medicine,
made her change her position, led her by the arm
here and there, washed and dressed her sores, removed the vermin, and would not allow himself
to be deterred even by what was most loathsome.

And for all this he asked no remuneration
whatsoever on the part of men; nay, he was far
more pleased when, in return for his zeal in tending the sick, he was allowed to suffer something,
occasions for which were, of course, not wanting.
Frequently the sick and dying in private houses
refused to see him, and at times he was received
with open insult. It is reported that many
times when, at night, he was called to dying persons living in the most remote back streets, he

was attacked, ill-treated, and robbed by the ruffians of the place, without his ever making a complaint against them.

23. The venerable servant of God *Maria Clotilda,* Queen of Sardinia (d. 1802), frequently went to see the nuns in the places where she made a stay, and conversed with them with great condescension, chiefly on pious subjects. If any of them were sick, she visited them in their poor cells. Her charity overcame all feelings of repugnance or fear of contagion; she encouraged and consoled them, exhorted them to patience, and if needful nursed them herself. She considered herself their inferior, convinced as she was that the wife of a prince is not to be compared with a spouse of Christ.

During the illness of her aunt, a royal princess, she rendered her the most lowly and abject services. She was never weary in exhorting her to be resigned, inspiring her with those holy aspirations so necessary for the last great journey. And if the king, out of regard for her own health, had not ordered her sometimes to retire, she would not have left the invalid for a single instant. Clotilda always obeyed without a word of reply, but the king was advised to allow the queen more liberty, as it was evident what violence it cost her to abstain from these works of charity. He consented, on condition, however, that the queen should retire as soon as she felt the least indisposition. This permission filled Clotilda with intense joy, being free, as she now felt herself, to follow the impulses of her loving heart. The agony of the princess lasted thirty hours, and during all this time Clotilda hardly ever left her bedside. She exercised the same charity towards her maid of honor. As soon as she heard of her illness she hastened to procure her all possible assistance. She visited and tended her with such zeal that the king said: "If I were to allow it, she would watch by her bedside the whole night." She sustained the invalid by her prayers and by her consoling words, and inspired her with holy sentiments. She embraced her, wiped off the perspiration, made her bed, and served her like a simple maid. During the three days that the mortal remains of the above-named princess were exposed the queen was obliged to suspend her visits to her maid of honor; but she sent other good souls to lend her assistance, and took care that she wanted nothing. She left the invalid in the care of the only maid of honor she retained, and ordered several persons to take turns in nursing her. One day the surgeon came to relieve the sufferer of an abscess. The queen was present; but her humble exterior and simple attire made him think she was the maid, whereupon he asked her to help him to make the bed, which she at once set about doing. When the invalid was about to undeceive the doctor, Clotilda silenced her by a sign. But what was the astonishment and dismay of the surgeon when a little while later he saw her leave the room accompanied by one of the officers of the court! When he learned that she was the queen he was not a little confused on account of his mistake.

24. *Blessed Clement Hofbauer* was a tender father of the sick, and it is impossible to describe with what love and solicitude he lavished spiritual assistance upon them. His first care was that all in the convent entrusted to him should appreciate at its true value, and turn to good account, the precious cross of sickness. He was also indefatigable in consoling and encouraging the sick nuns and confirming them in the love of the cross and resignation to the will of God.

In the infirmary of the convent there was an aged Sister who, being somewhat deranged in mind, was so peevish and impatient that she was a burden to the rest of the Community. Father Hofbauer used daily to visit her during her illness, but he never did so until he had picked a few flowers in the garden, which he gave to her. If there were no flowers, he brought her some other trifle, which caused her pleasure the whole day. Then he would begin to converse on household matters, as she took no interest in spiritual ones. Thus by degrees he won her affection and confidence. She was completely overcome by his inviting her to take a walk through the cloister and offering his arm to support her, as she walked only with great difficulty. So much love and sympathy worked an entire change in the poor Sister; she became patient and gay and was no longer a burden and a trouble to her infirmarians. When later on she was inclined to be irritable, it was sufficient to remind her of this walk and she became at once calm and cheerful.

He showed similar love to all the sick Sisters, especially when they drew near their death. At every hour of the day or night he was ready to assist them. Frequently he would watch through the whole night and bring holy communion to the sick shortly after midnight.

Father Hofbauer's love for the sick was, however, not confined to the convent only; it led him to beds of sickness wherever they might be, whether in the palaces of the rich, or in the hovels of the poor, or in the various hospitals of the town. No one could number the sick whom, during his stay at Vienna, he visited, consoled, and prepared for their last journey.

The servant of God never refused to go to the sick even at the dead of night, or to distant suburbs through rain, snow, or wind. To poor people he occasionally brought food and similar alms; and if necessary he took the place of an infirmarian. His exceeding love and affability easily won him the affection and confidence of all, and enabled him to snatch from the clutch of Satan many a dying sinner who already seemed the prey of hell. If he had to attend a sick-call of this kind, he used to say his rosary as he went along the road, and he also asked the nuns to pray that he might secure the wished-for result. Great was his joy when he could announce to the Sisters the happy news that a great sinner, who had not been to confession for twenty or thirty years, had been converted and had died the death of a penitent.

25. The venerable servant of God *Canon Cottolengo* when but a boy of five years old gave evident signs of his love for the sick. One day when he was measuring with a cord one room after the other, his mother asked him what he intended to do. " Dear mother," was the reply, " I want to see how many beds can be placed in this house; when I am grown up I should like to fill the whole house with sick people." A tear of emotion glistened in his mother's eye, while the child with great earnestness continued his work. In 1832 he founded at Turin the " Little Asylum of Divine Providence," which at the present day has obtained an extraordinary celebrity. It is, as it were, a small town within the large one; it shelters five thousand men and embraces within its precincts a church, a number of houses, courtyards, terraces, subterranean passages, etc. Two things especially characterized this apostle of charity. In the first place, he received no sick persons who could be sufficiently provided for in their own houses, as he declared that his establishment was first of all the property of those who were entirely destitute and forsaken. Secondly, he was determined that all the poor and sick should be treated with the best possible care. The beds were to be soft and comfortable, the food well prepared, the wine of the best sort. On Sundays and holidays he himself distributed fruit, cake, and sweetmeats to his sick. He used to say to the nursing

Sisters: " The sick must be as dear to us as the apple of our eye; therefore we give them all they wish, provided it is not hurtful. They are the masters of the house; let us serve them well, or else they have a right to put us outside the door." As for those who were suffering from any mental affliction, he desired them to be treated with consideration, and never would he allow words such as " madman," " maniac," etc., to be uttered in their presence. He called them his " good children," and placed them under the special patronage of the Holy Innocents. In spite of the heavy work with which he was burdened he led an exceedingly austere and mortified life. For a long time he had not in his establishment even a room for his own use; he was always to be found where he was most needed, and he slept on a chair in one of the wards. In consequence of the ill treatment that he met with from a wicked man on one of his nightly sick-calls in the year 1842, a pulmonary disease developed, which, combined with a chronic fever, soon put an end to his saintly life.

26. In the year 1863 *Father Damien de Veuster*, of the Congregation of the Most Sacred Hearts of Jesus and Mary, was sent to Oceania as a missionary. After the lapse of ten years he came to Molokai, one of the smaller of the Sandwich Islands. Its population consisted of three thousand lepers who had been sent there by the government of Hawaii. He then asked his superiors as a special favor to be allowed to remain with the unfortunate victims of this terrible malady. His

request was granted, and during the remaining sixteen years of his life the undaunted missionary indefatigably tended these poor lepers, who were literally rotting to death, and encouraged them by his fatherly consolations. Writing to his family and friends in Europe, he said he felt so happy in his office that no human consideration could induce him to separate himself from his beloved lepers. Nevertheless he was well aware that he would have to pay for his loving service with his own life. Four years before his death the first symptoms of leprosy appeared on his face, and from month to month, from week to week, he could discern the progress of the devastating evil which finally caused his limbs one after the other to drop from his body. But in spite of this decay the heroic man remained fearless, never losing his supernatural joy and serenity. At length, on the 15th of April, 1889, after having bidden a last farewell to the religious who had come to his assistance, he consummated his sacrifice and breathed his last, filled with heavenly peace and happiness.

27. In the Dutch possessions of Surinam (South America) we find another martyr of Christian charity, who is by no means inferior to the one just mentioned, namely, *Father John Bakker,* a Dutch Redemptorist (d. 1890). From 1866, that is to say, for twenty-four years, he devoted himself to the spiritual and bodily care of the lepers in that place. For ten whole years he himself suffered from leprosy, and the last months of

his life in particular were exceedingly tormenting. All his fingers had to be amputated, and the malady daily gained ground within him; yet notwithstanding his sufferings he continued tranquil and submissive to the will of God until the hour of his death.

PART II.

SICK-NURSING IN GENERAL.

CHAPTER I.

Consoling the Sick.

The first four chapters of this second part, are chiefly devoted to the consolation and instruction of invalids. They can be read to them, or made the subject of conversation.

To make the sick man comply with the loving designs of God, who sends his illness, it is above all of the greatest importance to make him realize that illness, with respect to the body, is undoubtedly an evil, but that it is of great profit to the soul if the sick man only knows how to make good use of it. Exhort him, therefore, to :

I. RECEIVE ILLNESS AS A LOVING DISPENSATION
OF GOD.

As health is numbered among the most precious of earthly goods, so illness is considered to be one of the greatest afflictions, especially when it is painful or of long duration, or when, the invalid

being at the same time stricken with poverty, it
is the cause of great want not only to himself but
also to his family. If we consider that without
God's will not a sparrow falleth from the tree, nor
a hair from our heads, we must be firmly convinced that whatsoever God destines for us
comes from His most wise and loving designs,
since for those who love God all things turn to
their good. "Can you," says St. Francis of Sales,
"find any one who loves you more than God?
He is your Father, otherwise Jesus would not have
ordered you to pray: 'Our Father, who art in
heaven.' Now as a child of such a father what
have you to fear? because without His will not a
hair falleth from your head. So, then, receive
with a filial, loving heart what God sends you with
a fatherly, loving heart."

1. Sometimes God sends us illness as a *salutary
medicine for the soul,* to make us amend our lives.
God willeth not the death of the sinner; on the
contrary, He tries all sorts of means to save his
soul. At one time He tries to allure him by prosperity and success; at another He speaks to his
heart interiorly by remorse of conscience, or else
exteriorly through the mouth of the priest, or
through frightful examples of His justice. But if
all this is of no avail, God makes use of stronger
and sharper expedients: He sends the sinner to
the school of sufferings, visiting him with crosses
and adversities; with a painful disease, for instance, that he may awake from his sinful slumber,
enter into his heart, and be converted. Christ,

our heavenly physician, acts like a surgeon who frequently orders bitter draughts, or endeavors to cure the sick man by burning and cauterizing his ulcers. He dispenses pain and suffering, not for the sake of tormenting us, but for healing us. Therefore also the Holy Spirit says: " A grievous sickness maketh the soul sober "; that is to say, brings the soul to a consciousness of its sinful state and a return to God (Ecclus. xxxi. 2).

When in health and free from suffering, man does not know how to appreciate these benefits of God; he thanks Him little or not at all; many even go so far as to forget their Lord and Creator and to squander their days in earthly enjoyments and sinful pleasures. The world with its enjoyments, and the flesh with its unrestrained propensities, get the mastery over them, and they would assuredly end in ruin if God did not take pity on them. For this purpose He sends them tribulation, visits them with illness, and deprives them of the things their hearts are clinging to. He confines them to a bed of sickness, takes from them their appetite, robs them of their sleep and the use of their limbs; thus showing them their misery and weakness, making known to them the vanity of this world and of its pleasures, and by this means humbling them. Now their eyes are opened, they see their sinful lives, and call upon God, who strikes only in order to heal.

It is true many will not acknowledge this. They complain and murmur against God's ordinances, give way to anger and impatience, or to pusilla-

nimity and faint-heartedness. They behave exactly like many invalids under the treatment of
the doctor when, perhaps, he prescribes bitter
medicines, forbids what they ask for, or increases
their sufferings by painful blisters, lancing and
searing, etc. But precisely because he wishes
well to the sick man and means to cure him, the
doctor does not take any account of his complaints. The good God does the same, and chastises with the scourge of illness, because He has at
heart the salvation of our soul. He frequently
prolongs the time of illness, increases its pains,
and withholds relief, only to bring man to a better
understanding and to save his soul.

Examples.

Gentilezza, a noble Roman lady, being proud of
her personal attractions, indulged not a little in
the enjoyments and vanities of this world. She
neglected her duties to her husband and children,
and gave herself up to pleasure without further
consideration. St. Frances of Rome, feeling compassion for her, endeavored by loving exhortations
to bring her to a better way of life. But she received her advice with nothing but scorn and
laughter. Frances then recommended her to God
in prayer, and one day said to her: " You laugh at
my warnings, as well as at those of your confessor; but you will soon learn that we cannot resist
God with impunity." Soon after Gentilezza fell
down one of the staircases in the palace, and was
taken up by her servants half dead; she had

broken her nose and cut her lips, and her state was declared hopeless by the doctors. In her prostrate, enfeebled state she thought only of the loss of her beauty, not of that of her soul. Then St. Frances drew near to her bed to comfort and assist her. With kind and gentle, yet earnest words, she described to the invalid her previous conduct, declaring that this accident was a punishment sent by God's fatherly mercy to lead her back from the paths of perdition and induce her to repent and do penance. Then Gentilezza, entering into herself, perceived the danger of her soul, and was convinced that God had indeed sent her this chastisement, and that she had deserved a far greater punishment. She bore with resignation the pains of her illness, and on being restored to health she became one of the holiest and most exemplary women of Rome.

St. Ignatius of Loyola up to his twenty-ninth year was a brave soldier but an indifferent Christian. At the siege of Pampeluna, one of his legs having been shattered by a cannon-ball, he fell into the hands of one of his enemies, who on account of his valor treated him with courtesy and had him transported to his own castle of Loyola. He had to keep his bed for some time and suffered intense pain. In order to divert his mind, he asked for some romances; but no such books were to be found in the castle, only "The Life of Jesus Christ" and "The Legends of the Saints." At first he read them with the greatest indifference, simply to while away the long and tedious hours;

but before long he was so much affected by their contents that he was filled with the greatest admiration of the examples of heroic virtue before his eyes. At length he was so deeply impressed that he determined to leave the world and henceforth to serve God alone. Seized with a salutary fear when he looked into the depths of his soul, so disfigured by his sins, he began a new life and suffered with cheerfulness and resignation the bodily pains which the Lord had sent him for the salvation of his soul.

St. Jerome relates how a noble Roman lady, of the name of *Blasilla,* who had formerly lived only for the world, was by sickness led to God. " Behold our Blasilla," writes the saint, " who used to stand nearly the whole day before the glass, curling her hair, and doing nothing but indulge her vanity. The Lord has visited her with a thirty days' fever and thrown her into a crucible of suffering. And see, now she no longer stands before the mirror, but before Jesus Christ, the mirror of the soul, and prays; she, who formerly lived only for the world and its pleasures, is now removed far from the perishable joys of this life; she rises early, hastens to prayer, and spends her days in good works; she, who was once a scandal to others, now attracts many to sing the praises of God; she, who formerly through vanity was afraid of soiling her dress, now kneels on the bare ground in prayer; she, who formerly found no time to think of God and look up to Him, now, after having been enlightened by illness, takes her greatest delight in being alone with Jesus Christ."

2. *Illness is sometimes a paternal chastisement of God, that thereby we may do penance for our sins.* When God visits us with a painful illness, we frequently behave no better than children. We complain, lament, murmur, and even give vent to our feelings by impatient words; we do not realize that it is God's fatherly hand which chastises us, nor think of His merciful designs in our regard. We feel indeed that we have deserved punishment, and perhaps we say to ourselves: "How shall I encounter the rigorous judgments of God ? What a severe punishment have I not to expect from Him !" But as to penance, we are too cowardly and faint-hearted to do it; we will not punish ourselves. Now, since we do not do it, God does it Himself through the compassion He has for us. He sends us some accident, affliction, or disease, giving us thereby an opportunity to expiate in some measure the faults we have committed. If, therefore, we bear the chastisements of God in a true spirit of penance, with patience, humility, and resignation, we shall reap great consolation in the day of retribution.

Writing on this subject, St. Alphonsus, doctor of the Church, says: "If, dear Christian soul, you must own to yourself that you have offended God, and if nevertheless you wish to obtain everlasting life, you must rejoice when God sends you sufferings." "Sin," says St. Chrysostom, "is an ulcer of the soul; if no adversity comes to make it discharge the poison, the soul is lost." Oh, how much to be pitied is the sinner who is not punished in this life for his misdeeds! For this reason you must return thanks to God for visiting you with sufferings; it is a sign that He loves you and holds you as His child." "Whom the Lord loveth He chastiseth; and He scourgeth every son whom He receiveth" (Heb. xii. 6). According to this, St. Augustine says: "If it is well with you, recognize the Father who caresses you; if you have to suffer, recognize the Father who chastises you." "How much, on the other hand, are you to be pitied," he adds, "if God, in spite of your sins, spares you the rod of correction on earth!" When, therefore, you are afflicted with tribulation, do not say that God has forgotten you; say rather you have forgotten your sins. He who has offended God must pray with St. Bonaventure: "Hasten, O Lord, hasten and wound Thy servants with the wounds of love and salvation, that we may not be struck by the wounds of wrath and of eternal death." God sends us sufferings not to ruin but to save us, and it is our own fault if we do not make good use of them. "Never," says St. Bernard, "is God more angry than when He does not frown on the sinner and chastise him." Hence the saint prayed: "I beseech Thee, O Lord, show Thyself a Father of mercy to me; that is to say, vouchsafe to punish me for my sins here below, in order to preserve me from everlasting punishment." "When, therefore," concludes St. Alphonsus, "God visits you with illness, humble yourself and say with the good thief: 'We indeed justly; for we receive the due reward of our deeds' (Luke xxiii. 41). Lord, I have deserved this cross, because I have offended Thee. Humble yourself, then, and be of good heart; for if God chastises you in this world, it is a sign that He means to spare you everlasting punishments hereafter."

Examples.

St. Stephen the hermit suffered so much from a terrible disease that a surgeon had to cut off his rotting flesh. While the bystanders, filled with compassion, condoled with him in his sufferings, he said: " My children, whatever God does is done with a good intention. Let us suffer and combat as long as we are in this world. Better is it to be chastised by transitory pain than to endure pains which have no end."

A man who employed his riches only in pomp, luxury, and costly banquets fell dangerously ill. His relatives recommended him to the prayers of *St. Francis of Sales,* who sent him a message bidding him have confidence, adding that his illness was not for death, but for the greater glory of God. He told him that in future he should amend his life in order that nothing worse might befall him. Contrary to all expectation the sick man recovered, and as soon as he was able he hastened to church to return thanks to God for having restored his health; he then visited the holy bishop to thank him for his intercession. " See, my

dear friend," said St. Francis, " the divine justice
frequently sends us in mercy such like evils, that
we, who do not do penance of our own accord,
may in this manner be forced to do it. Happy he
who knows how to avail himself of it and makes
a virtue of necessity! God does not show such
favor to every one; not to all does He manifest
His judgments with such great benignity. Return thanks to Him for this rod of paternal correction, with which He in His mercy has chastised
you. It was good for you to have been humbled
a little; it was to make you acknowledge and
adore His just decrees."

For many years *St. Vincent of Paul* suffered the
most violent pains without ever uttering any complaint. When they were more than usually intense he would look up to his crucifix and say :
" What I suffer is very little compared with what
I deserve to suffer and what Christ has suffered for
my sake." One day one of his religious brothers,
on seeing his legs all swollen and covered with
ulcers, was moved with compassion and exclaimed:
" Truly your pain must be insupportable ! "
" How can you," interrupted the saint, " how can
you call the work of God insupportable, because
He causes a miserable sinner to suffer ? May God
forgive you these words ! This is not the manner
of speaking in the school of Christ. Is it not just
that the guilty should suffer and be chastised ?
Has not the Lord a right to do with us what He
pleases ? "

3. *Illness is a touchstone of virtue as well as a*

means of perfection. St. Alphonsus writes on this subject as follows: " ' There are many,' says the Wise Man, ' who are friends in time of prosperity, but who abandon their friend when misfortune befalls him.' Many a one is a friend only as long as he thinks it to be good, but in the day of tribulation he keeps aloof; and yet the most certain proof of true affection consists in suffering willingly for one's friend. Therefore the most pleasing sacrifice we can offer to God is to embrace willingly whatever cross He sends. Charity is patient; it beareth all things; it readily beareth exterior crosses, such as the loss of health, of goods, of honor, of relatives and friends, as also interior ones: anxieties, temptations, pain, and spiritual aridity. Virtue is tried by patience; therefore those who write the lives of the saints endeavor to give a prominent place to their patience in adversity. The devil tempts us for the sake of plunging us into ruin; God, on the other hand, tempts us in order to try our patience. Like gold in the furnace He tries them; that is to say, as gold is tried by means of fire, so does God put to the test the love of His servants by the fire of adversity. If, therefore, a soul has many contradictions to suffer, it is a sign that God loves her, as the angel assured Tobias: ' Because thou wast acceptable to God, it was necessary that temptation should prove thee ' (xii. 13). St. Chrysostom says : ' If the Lord gives any one the opportunity of suffering much, He shows him a greater favor than if He were to give him the power of raising the dead to life; for if we work miracles, we are the debtors of God; but if we suffer with patience, God becomes, as it were, our debtor.' 'Illness,' says St. Bernard, 'is the touchstone of our dispositions and proves whether they are genuine gold or only tinsel. Many are cheerful, patient, and devout as long as they enjoy good health; but when they are visited by sickness they act as though they were quite inconsolable; they are impatient towards everybody, even to those who assist them through charity; they fret at the least pain, the most trifling inconvenience; they have complaints to make against every one— against the physician, their parents, their attendants. Then it clearly appears that what was supposed to be gold is only copper.'" Thus far St. Alphonsus.

Gold and silver are not only proved, but also cleansed in the fire; in like manner, virtues are not only tried in the crucible of affliction, but also purified and perfected. By what means do we show to God that we love Him truly and above all things? In what do true virtue and perfection consist? All theologians assure us that our perfection does not consist in a number of prayers or penances, etc., but in the perfect accomplishment of the divine will; in other words, in our seeking and willing in all things nothing but what God wills, so that in all the vicissitudes of life, in health as well as in sickness, we say with the same resignation and loyalty: "Thy will be done on earth as it is in heaven." "Suffering," says St. Thomas of Villanova, "reveals the hidden power of endurance of a just man. The grain of pepper or mustard does not manifest its interior power until it is broken and crushed." Afflictions, calamities, and sufferings, among which illness holds a prominent place, are not only trials sent by God, but they purify and refine the soul as fire purifies and refines gold and silver. These metals when taken from the mine are still mixed with dross, which it requires the action of fire to remove. So the souls of virtuous men are often hampered with a variety of faults and imperfections highly displeasing in the eyes of God. Therefore He sends them sufferings and pains, in order to cleanse and make them pleasing in His sight. "And I will bring them through the fire, and will refine them as silver is refined," says the Lord through the prophet Zacharias, " and I will try them as gold is tried " (xiii. 9).

Examples.

St. Henry, Emperor of Germany, lying sick of a painful malady, did not complain, but said : " God sends us bodily disease in order to preserve us in humility; His chastisements are so many tokens of His love for us."

St. John Capistran said one day to a sick man: " You are perhaps surprised, but I rejoice at your illness. Why should I grieve at what God sends you ? Through illness God means to test your

patience; for He smites His elect only in order
to heal them."

St. Vincent of Paul was constantly ill. Violent
and continual fevers racked him day and night.
Asthma, as well as pains in his head and stomach,
often made him suffer tortures. A swelling on his
leg forced him to use a stick, and a painful sore-
ness of the eyes almost deprived him of sight.
Two years before his death ulcers formed on his
ankle and obliged him to use crutches. At last
he was confined to an armchair, suffering day
and night the most acute pain without either
rest or relief, nay, even without being able to
move. But all these sufferings did not make him
utter a single complaint, nor did his cheerfulness
and affability towards everybody diminish in the
least. Like a hero he withstood the trial sent to
him by God. In this trying state he was often
heard to praise and bless the Lord. " It is true," he
said one day to his brothers in religion, " the state
of illness is painful and seems unbearable to nature, but for all that it is one of the most cogent
means which God makes use of to disengage our
heart from all affection to sin, and to enrich us
with innumerable graces. O my Saviour, who
didst suffer so much and die to redeem us, and to
show us how agreeable in the sight of God and
how expedient for our sanctification suffering is:
grant us the grace to esteem at its true value the
great good and the hidden treasure that is to be
found in sickness ! "

4. *Illness is a source of merits.* St. Alphonsus,

doctor of the Church, says: " In your illness console yourself with the hope of heaven." Blessed Joseph Calasanctius says: " All trouble must be deemed as trifling to gain heaven." And before him the Apostle says: " For I reckon, that the sufferings of this time are not worthy to be compared with the glory to come, that shall be revealed in us " (Rom. viii. 18).

It would be but a small thing if we had to endure all the sufferings of this world in order to be allowed to enjoy for only one instant the delights of heaven. With how much reason, then, should we embrace with joy whatever cross God lays upon us, knowing as we do that the short-lived sufferings of this life yield everlasting bliss for heaven ! " For that which is at present momentary and light of our tribulation, worketh for us above measure exceedingly an eternal weight of glory " (2 Cor. iv. 17). Instead of being troubled, therefore, we ought to rejoice with all our hearts if God visits us with sufferings on this earth. He who enters eternity laden with the greatest store of merits will also reap the greatest reward; and this is the reason why God sends us adversities here below. Virtues which are the source of merit are only acquired by practice. Now, a person who frequently undergoes periods of suffering and has to encounter many humiliations finds opportunity for practising numerous acts of patience. Therefore St. James encourages us, saying: " Blessed is the man that endureth temptation : for when he hath been proved," that is to

say, when he has stood the trial, " he shall receive
the crown of life " (James i. 12). Animated by
this thought, St. Agapitus, a youth of fifteen, displayed a wonderful heroism while suffering the
pangs of martyrdom. The tyrant having caused
burning coals to be placed on his head, the young
martyr said: " It is truly a little thing that this
head should be burned which in heaven is to be
crowned with splendor." The same thought
brought the following words into the mouth of holy
Job: " If we have received good things at the hand
of God, why should we not receive evil ? " (ii. 10.)
He meant to say : If we have received perishable
goods with joy from the Lord, why should we not
receive with still greater joy passing evils, which
procure us the everlasting joys of heaven ? And
again it was this thought which made St. Francis
say: " The good I expect is so great that every
pain is a pleasure to me." In a word, the saints
rejoice when they have to suffer tribulation here
on earth, and in a certain measure are grieved
when they are in prosperity.

The sick when they see their last hour drawing
near should above all resign themselves to death,
and to whatever kind of death God may send them.
After all, what is life but an unceasing storm
which continually exposes us to the danger of
being lost forever ? St. Aloysius, although dying
in the prime of life, joyfully accepted death, saying: " Now, because I hope I am in the grace of
God, and not knowing what may befall me hereafter, I am willing to die, provided it pleases God

to call me hence." "But," you will say, "Aloysius was a saint, and I am a sinner." Listen to what Blessed John of Avila tells you in answer: "If we find ourselves in good dispositions, though only moderately good, we ought to desire death, in order to escape the danger of losing the grace of God, to which we are continually exposed here on earth. How desirable is it through death to obtain the certainty of never losing God!" "But," you reply, "up to the present I have not gained any merit; I should like to live longer, in order to do some good before I die." But who tells you that in a prolonged life you will not become worse than before? that you will not fall into grievous sin and be lost? Upon earth no one lives without sin, at least not without venial sin. The thought of this caused St. Bernard to say: "Why do we ask to live, since the longer we live the more we offend God?" Besides, if we love God, we must long to enjoy His presence in heaven; yet if death does not open the gate for us, we cannot enter this blessed home. Therefore, St. Augustine, inflamed by the love of God, exclaimed: "Lord, let me die, that I may behold Thee!"

Examples.

Father Balthasar Alvarez was allowed one day to behold the great glory which God had prepared for a nun on account of her patient endurance of an illness; and he assures us that this pious religious had obtained more merits during the eight months of her illness than other zealous nuns in the course of several years.

St. Lidwina saw an exceedingly brilliant but unfinished crown, and understood that it was destined for herself; wishing the crown to be finished she asked God to increase her sufferings. Her supplications were heard, and God allowed soldiers to come to her, who not only overwhelmed her with abuse, but also grievously illtreated her. Then an angel appeared, and, showing her the finished crown, said that these last sufferings had supplied the precious stones that had been wanting. Soon after she went to reap her reward in heaven.

St. Regina, Virgin, while lying in a dungeon, with her body all lacerated by scourging, saw a high cross reaching from earth to heaven, with a dove on the top holding a wreath in its bill. At the same time she heard these words: " Your sufferings will be a ladder to heaven." But how are sufferings and pain a ladder to heaven ? They become a ladder by the way the sufferer bears them. The ladder on which a person ascends must stand firmly on the ground; its two arms must be strong, its steps solid. The ground on which this ladder to heaven must stand is the firm, immutable faith that all sorrows and sufferings come from God, and that He sends them for our good. The two arms of the ladder are love and confidence. The sick man must suffer for love of God, and have a firm confidence that God will grant him requisite strength to bear his cross and that he will never be forsaken. By the steps are signified acknowledgment of our sinfulness, our spirit of penance, our humility, and our calm resignation to and union with the divine will. The sufferer who stands firm in his belief of the almighty providence of God, and clings to Him by the two arms of love and confidence, will safely ascend to heaven, where his crown awaits him.

Being near death, *St. Rose of Lima* burst into tears. When asked the reason, she answered : " I do not weep because I have to leave the earth; this in truth gives me the least sorrow; but I weep because I have not suffered enough to deserve heaven."

II. BEAR ILLNESS WITH RESIGNATION TO THE WILL OF GOD.

(Taken from the writings of St. Alphonsus.)

He who wishes to please God must long for opportunities of doing His good pleasure; therefore pious Christians look upon these providential dispensations which the world calls misfortunes as graces, and so much the greater graces as they are the more painful and hard to bear. Sick persons who have to suffer much and are not wholly resigned to the will of God are indeed greatly to be pitied, not exactly because they suffer, but because they do not know how to appreciate the great treasures which God offers them by means of suffering. Nay, they convert into a poison what is sent them as a remedy, for, according to the words of the Wise Man, " Bodily ailments are the most efficacious means of healing the evils of the soul."

He, on the contrary, who in time of adversity and pain resigns himself to the will of God speeds on, as Father Balthasar Alvarez says, with rapid steps towards union with God. This is what the Lord Himself revealed to St. Gertrude, saying to her that whenever He beheld any one in affliction He felt drawn towards him, and it gave Him the greatest delight to be with the sick and afflicted. If, therefore, we suffer from some illness, we can, nay, we ought to make use of the remedies prescribed by the doctor, because God so wills it; but having done this, we must resign ourselves entirely to the will of God. We may also ask Him for health, with the view of employing it in His service, at the same time leaving ourselves entirely in His hands, that He may do with us what He pleases: these are the best means to regain health. He who in his prayers seeks only himself instead of seeking God is not heard, while he who in his pleadings has only God and His holy will in view is always heard. " I sought the Lord, and He heard me " (Ps. xxxiii. 5). What a powerful remedy for all sorts of maladies we possess in the words: " Lord, Thy will be done " ! Therefore when attacked by illness abandon yourself entirely to the will of God, ready to suffer whatever He may send you; be united to Jesus on the cross, and do not desire to descend from it ere it pleases Him that you should do so; show yourself ready even to die, if such be His holy will.   Always have your crucified Saviour before your eyes; you will assuredly suffer with far greater patience when you consider how trifling your pains are compared with those which Jesus Christ suffered for the love of you.

"But," many a sick person objects, "I suffer so much, and may I not even complain or communicate to others what I suffer ?"   You are not forbidden to make your pains known to others when they are violent; but if they are slight, it is a weakness to complain to everybody and seek for sympathy.   If the remedies used do not prove efficacious, you must practise patience and resign yourself entirely to the will of God.   "If we knew," says St. Vincent of Paul, "what a valuable treasure is hidden in illness, we would accept it joyfully as the greatest of benefits."   The saint therefore bore without a shadow of complaint the acute sufferings which were caused by his constant infirmities, and which were so great that often, neither by day nor by night, did he find any rest; nay, he was always so cheerful that it seemed as if he had nothing at all to endure.   Oh, how edifying it is when we see one in illness continue calm and resigned !

This was the case with St. Francis of Sales, who when ill simply explained his ailment to the physician, whom he obeyed by taking the remedies prescribed, however distasteful they might be; and having done this he remained perfectly calm, without the least complaint.   What a

splendid example for those who in the slightest
indispositions are continually lamenting and wishing to have the sympathy of their relatives and
friends ! " Learn how to suffer for the love of
God," said St. Teresa, " and do not wish that
every one should know it." By a special grace,
Blessed Father Louis of Ponte was afflicted one
Good Friday with so many bodily sufferings that
every part of his body had a special torture to endure. He made this known to one of his friends,
but hardly had he uttered the words when he
regretted it so much that he made a vow never
again to confide to others what he might have to
suffer. I said just now " by a special grace," for
the saints regard as favors the illnesses and tribulations which God sends them.

Many an invalid in his impatience exclaims :
" Where is charity to be found ? See how they
forget me, leaving me to lie on this bed of pain ! "
Poor sick man, I pity you, not on account of your
illness, but on account of your want of patience,
which makes you doubly ill, ill in body and ill in
soul. Others have forgotten you; but you have
forgotten Jesus Christ, who, abandoned by all,
died on the cross for your sake. Why do you complain of this one or that one ? Blame yourself for
having so little love for your divine Saviour, and
in consequence so little patience. To a pious
woman who was lying ill, tortured by violent pain,
a crucifix was given, and she was at the same time
advised to beseech Our Lord to free her from her
pain. " How can you expect me to desire to de-

scend from the cross," she answered, "while I hold my crucified Saviour in my hands ? Willingly I suffer for the love of Him who for the love of me wished to suffer much greater pains than mine." Jesus Christ Himself one day said the same to St. Teresa when she was ill and suffering great pain. He appeared to her all covered with wounds, saying : " Behold these wounds, My daughter ; your pains will never be as great as Mine." Therefore the saint when suffering from any disease used to say: " When I consider in how many ways Our Saviour suffered, He who was perfectly innocent, I do not know how I could complain of my sufferings." " Many," says Salvian, " would never arrive at sanctity if they had good health." In fact, we read of the saints that nearly all of them were subject to a variety of illnesses. " Therefore," Salvian adds, " those who have consecrated themselves to the love of Christ are often ill, and wish to be ill."

Another says: " I do not complain of being ill; but I am sorry for not being able to go to church, to receive holy communion, to pray, and for being a burden to others." Allow me to make answer severally to each of these grievances. Tell me why you would go to church and receive holy communion ? To please God, is it not ? Well, but if it is now pleasing to God that you should not go to church and not receive holy communion, but that you should lie on a bed of pain, what reason have you to grieve ? Only listen to what Blessed John of Avila wrote one day to a sick priest: "My dear friend, do not consider now what you would do if you were in health, but be content to be ill as long as it pleases God. If you seek the will of God, what can it matter to you whether you are ill or in good health?" St. Francis of Sales asserts that we serve God better by suffering than by working. But you say you cannot pray. Why can you not pray? I grant that you cannot apply yourself to meditation, but what prevents you from turning your eyes upon Jesus crucified and offering to Him the pains you suffer? When at the height of your sufferings your best prayer is to resign yourself to the will of God, unite your pains with those of Jesus Christ, and offer them as a sacrifice to God. This is what St. Vincent of Paul did when he was lying prostrated by illness. He quietly put himself in the presence of God without over-exerting himself to fix his attention, but being content from time to time to make an act of love, of confidence, of thanksgiving, or of resignation, especially when his pains grew more intense. St. Francis of Sales said: "Tribulations in themselves are horrible; considered as being the will of God they give joy and delight." Finally, you say, you cannot work in this state; you are a burden to others. But in the same measure as you submit to the will of God you must presuppose the same of others; they see well enough that it is not through your own fault that you have become a burden to them, but because God will have it so. All such wishes and complaints do not spring from the love of God, but from self-love; we would fain serve God, not as it pleases Him, but as it pleases us.

Examples.

St. Mary Magdalen of Pazzi had to endure for several years the greatest pains; in consequence of vomiting blood she was reduced to such a degree of weakness that the physician wondered how so enfeebled a body could bear such sufferings. Nevertheless, through the power of God, who wished to assuage her thirst for suffering, she continued to live several years, all the while finding no rest but in God, her Saviour. With deep interior peace she said to Him: "If Thou, O Lord, dost not grant me strength and help, my body cannot bear so much." However trying and manifold her sufferings might be, her patience and resignation to the will of God were so great that she frequently raised her eyes to heaven, thanking Him that He prolonged her life to be able to suffer more; at the same time offering herself as a victim to the divine Majesty, she exclaimed: "Lord, if it is Thy good pleasure that I should be confined to this bed until the Last Day, let Thy will be done." She taught the following beautiful lesson to one of her sisters in religion who was struck by her admirable resignation: "When you have sufferings, take good care not to separate them from their origin, which is the will of God; otherwise they will be an insupportable burden to you." Being one day asked by her confessor if her sufferings were great, the saint answered: "Not one limb of my body is without pain, but in my heart I find great rest, as it is the will of God."

Laurence of the Resurrection, a lay Brother of the Carmelite Order, was so content in his sufferings that his very face reflected his interior joy. Being asked if he had nothing to suffer, because he invariably looked so joyful, he replied: "Oh, yes, I do suffer; my side causes me great pain, yet I am happy." "But, dear Brother," he was further asked, "if it were God's will that you should bear these pains ten years longer, would you then be contented?" "Yes," was the reply, "not only so many years, but if it pleased God that I should bear these pains until the Day of Judgment, I would gladly resign myself to them, in hopes that God would grant me the grace to bear all for His sake."

In his old age *St. Alphonsus* had a severe attack of illness which lasted longer than a year, and was accompanied by a total absence of sleep. "I would fain have slept a little," he would sometimes say, "but since God wills it not, neither do I."

We read in the life of *St. Thomas of Canterbury,* Archbishop and Martyr, that a certain sick man made a pilgrimage to his tomb in order to regain health through his intercession. He returned home in perfect health and full of joy. On the following Sunday or feast-day he assisted at Mass, and heard a sermon in which the preacher explained how a Christian has to pray; how his petitions should always be accompanied by an act of resignation to the will of God, such as: "Lord, give me this or that; restore my health, if it be Thy holy will and good for my salvation." Without delay the man returned to the tomb of St. Thomas of Canterbury, where he implored God that His holy will alone should be accomplished in him, and in case health should not be good for him he asked fervently for a return of ill health. This petition was granted; and the man was pleased, because he saw that thus he would arrive sooner at eternal bliss.

III. ENDEAVOR TO SUFFER ILLNESS JOYFULLY.

(Taken from the writings of St. Alphonsus.)

Whether we will or will not, all of us must suffer; so, then, let us try to suffer *meritoriously*, that is to say, *patiently*. Patience is a shield which protects us against all the tribulations entailed by persecutions, illnesses, losses, and other evils. Without this shield we are a prey to all those evils. Let us, then, first of all determine to beseech God to give us patience, for we shall not obtain this great grace unless we desire it. If we meet with some contradiction, let us do violence to ourselves, so as not to break out into impatient words or complaints: a fire soon dies out when access of air is prevented. Besides, before long we shall taste the fruits of victory. "To him who overcomes I will give a hidden manna." If in suffering and adversity we do violence to ourselves and willingly embrace the cross God sends us, He will give us great consolation, even in the midst of our tribulation—a consolation which, it is true, is hidden from worldly men, but which is well known to those who love Jesus Christ. " To suffer tribulation with a good conscience renders a person more happy than to enjoy all sorts of delights with a bad conscience."

There is *no cross* for him who is determined to suffer for God; or rather such a one *rejoices in his sufferings.* Let us peruse the lives of the saints, and we shall see how much they loved suffering.

St. Gertrude said suffering gave her so much joy that no time was more trying for her than when she had nothing to suffer. St. Teresa declares that she could not live without suffering, for which reason she frequently exclaimed: " Either suffer or die."

St. Mary Magdalen of Pazzi went still further, taking for her motto: " Suffer and not die."

" Torment me as much as you please," said St. Procopius the martyr, to the tyrant who kept inflicting fresh tortures upon him, " but do not forget that he who loves Jesus Christ desires nothing more ardently than to suffer for the love of Him."

Being threatened with a cruel death if he refused to deny his divine Master, St. Gordius answered: " I am sorry I can die but once for Jesus Christ, my Saviour " ; whereupon he went to meet his death with undaunted courage.

Charles Spinola wrote from his prison, where

he experienced great suffering : " Oh, how sweet it is to suffer for Jesus Christ ! I have already heard my sentence; I beseech you, thank the divine Goodness for the great grace He grants me ! " And he signed himself: " Charles Spinola, sentenced to death for the love of Jesus Christ." Shortly after he was roasted alive. When tied to the stake, he is said to have chanted the psalm: " Praise the Lord, all ye nations," and so singing he gave up the ghost.

" But," some one may ask, " how could the holy martyrs suffer so joyfully ? Were they not flesh and blood as we are, or had God rendered them insensible to pain ? " St. Bernard answers: " It was not insensibility but the love of Jesus Christ which made them suffer with such great patience and joy. Pain was not wanting, but they overcame and despised it through the love of their divine Master." A great servant of God, Hippolytus Durazzo, of the Society of Jesus, said : " Whatever God may cost us, we never buy Him too dearly." " He who does not know how to suffer for Jesus Christ," said Blessed Joseph Calasanctius, " does not know how to win Jesus Christ." Souls who understand the language of love find in the cross the fulfilment of all their wishes; that is to say, they please God if they willingly embrace it.

How is it possible to look at the crucifix and to behold a God who died in an ocean of pain and contempt, without bearing not only patiently but even embracing joyfully all and every suffering for His love ! St. Mary Magdalen of Pazzi said: "Every pain, however great it may be, becomes sweet if we contemplate Jesus on the cross." The learned Justus Lipsius having once great pain to endure, one of the bystanders encouraged him to patience, pointing out to him the example of some pagan philosophers; but the sufferer, lifting up his eyes to the crucifix, said: "Here is true patience !" He meant to say, the example of a God who suffered so much for our love is a sufficient motive for us to suffer every pain for His love. "He who loves Jesus crucified," says St. Bernard, "also loves pain and ignominy."

Examples.

Several months before his death *Blessed Peter Canisius* had the most acute pains to endure. His nerves were so unstrung that the least touch occasioned him the most violent suffering; he could neither sit nor lie without pain. One day the Brother Infirmarian said to him: "Dear Father, can you not ask Our Lord to send you some relief in your sufferings ?" Blessed Canisius replied: "Let us leave this good Master to rule; He knows better than we do what is needful ; for the many years that I have had the honor to serve Him I have always given myself up entirely to His loving providence, and have found this practice too advantageous to my soul to withdraw from it for the short time that remains for me to live."

The venerable servant of God *Bartholomew*, Archbishop of Braga, had such violent pains to endure that he frequently fell into a swoon. However, all the while he did not cease to praise God and to thank Him for His many graces. In the words of St. Fulgentius, he frequently used to exclaim: " Lord, grant me patience now, and mercy hereafter ! " Then he often recalled to his memory Pope Pius V., who, in the most excruciating sufferings, caused by stone, always repeated the prayer: " Lord, augment the pain, but also increase my patience."

Tortured by a most painful attack of the gout, *Louis de Ponte, S.J.*, asked for an increase of pain, and this was granted. For several months he could not leave his room, being compelled to use crutches in order to avoid touching the ground with his feet. Besides, he suffered from most painful complaints of the abdomen; his stomach was so weak that it did not retain any food, but rejected everything, and this was the cause of unspeakable pain to him. But the most trying of all were the pains of his chest, which frequently impeded his breathing and endangered his life. These and other sufferings did he bear with unshaken patience for the space of thirty-five years, until his death. His love for Jesus crucified, however, rendered his sufferings so sweet that he always asked for more. When one day a new remedy was recommended to him, he said: " It may be good, but I declare I do not wish to recover, unless it be for the greater glory of God."

For many years he had prayed that the fresh water which was his only relief might also become insipid to him. His prayer was heard. It went so far that he was absolutely forbidden to drink any more fresh water, but only that which was lukewarm. And frequently, owing to the negligence of the infirmarian, even this was not offered him. He kept silence, endured the privation, and made a sacrifice of it to God.

Consoling Thoughts for the Sick.

I. FROM HOLY SCRIPTURE.

" Through many tribulations we must enter into the kingdom of God " (Acts xiv. 21).

" Whom the Lord loveth, He chastiseth: and He scourgeth every son whom He receiveth " (Heb. xii. 6).

" Son, take all that shall be brought upon thee: and in thy sorrow endure, and in thy humiliation keep patience : For gold and silver are tried in the fire, but acceptable men in the furnace of humiliation " (Ecclus. ii. 4, 5).

" But God forbid that I should glory, save in the cross of Our Lord Jesus Christ " (Gal. vi. 14).

" The sufferings of this time are not worthy to be compared with the glory to come, that shall be revealed in us " (Rom. viii. 18).

" If we suffer with Him, we may be also glorified with Him " (Rom. viii. 17).

" And God shall wipe away all tears from their

eyes: and death shall be no more, nor mourning, nor crying, nor sorrow shall be any more, for the former things are passed away " (Apoc. xxi. 4).

" Eye hath not seen, nor ear heard, neither hath it entered into the heart of man, what things God hath prepared for them that love Him " (1 Cor. ii. 9).

" That which is at present momentary and light of our tribulation, worketh for us above measure exceedingly an eternal weight of glory " (2 Cor. iv. 17).

" Your sorrow shall be turned into joy . . . and your joy no man shall take from you " (John xvi. 20, 22).

" He that shall persevere to the end, he shall be saved " (Matt. xxiv. 13).

" Be thou faithful unto death, and I will give thee the crown of life " (Apoc. ii. 10).

" To him that shall overcome, I will give to sit with Me in My throne " (Apoc. iii. 21).

" Do not lose your confidence, which hath a great reward. For patience is necessary for you; that doing the will of God, you may receive the promise " (Heb. x. 35, 36).

" They that sow in tears shall reap in joy. Going they went and wept, casting their seeds. But coming they shall come with joyfulness, carrying their sheaves " (Ps. cxxv. 5–7).

" Blessed is the man that endureth temptation: for when he hath been proved, he shall receive the crown of life, which God hath promised to them that love Him " (James i. 12).

II. SAYINGS OF THE SAINTS.

" Every pain appears trifling to him who thinks that he has deserved hell " (St. Alphonsus).

" The best prayer in illness is to resign one's self to the will of God " (St. Alphonsus).

" How many bad persons are in health for whose salvation it would be better if they were ill ! " (St. Augustine.)

" God is served better by suffering than by work " (St. Francis of Sales).

" If you keep the greatness of your reward in view, everything you suffer will appear light to you; for in order to obtain everlasting rest, it is but just that we should work forever; and in order to win everlasting bliss, that we should suffer forever " (St. Augustine).

" Consider and contrast one with the other—the work and the tribulation, the glory and the reward. Compare what is momentary with what is eternal, what is light with what is important. The work you have, the tribulation you suffer, is momentary; but the glory which is waiting for you is eternal. Light and trifling is what you suffer; great and important is what you expect " (St. Peter Damian).

" So great is the delight of the glory to come that were one single drop of it to fall into hell it would change all its torments into beatitude " (St. Augustine).

" Better is it to suffer pain and to go to heaven

than to remain in health and to be damned" (St. Bernard).

"The good I expect is so great that every suffering is pleasant to me" (St. Francis of Assisi).

"If we look for what is sweet, we must necessarily first bear what is bitter" (St. Isidore).

"As on earth there is no one to be found who is immortal, so in like manner not one is to be found who is entirely without tribulation" (St. John Chrysostom).

"As the ring is a sign of nuptials, so are sufferings, if endured for the love of God, the surest sign of divine election, and are, as it were, the marriage of the soul with God" (words of Christ to St. Gertrude).

"One single 'Thanks be to God!' spoken in time of adversity is worth more than a thousand thanksgivings at a time when everything goes according to our wishes" (Blessed John of Avila).

"One ounce of the cross outweighs a thousand pounds of prayer. To spend one day fixed to the cross is better than a hundred years spent in other spiritual exercises. To be one instant on the cross is better than to taste the delights of paradise" (Venerable Sister Victoria Angelini, Servite nun).

III. MAXIMS.

The way of the cross leads to heaven.

Suffering will not last always; impatience makes it worse.

Thou complainest of God, when God has so much reason to complain of thee.

Silence, silence! Lord, Thy will—let it be accomplished in me! Amen! Amen!

And Thy name—let it be praised there and here.

The cross is the way to heaven, if thou art patient in thy crosses.

If a sorrow comes to thee, keep still and ask what it wants of thee; Eternal Love sends it to thee not only that thou mayest weep.

God is nothing but love and mercy; therefore, soul, hope patiently.

Everything as God wills; let everything be referred to Him.

He who confides in God like a child is established on a firm foundation.

O death, O death, how sweet thou art! Thou bringest me to the Lord in paradise.

O gentle death, make haste and come quickly to me, that I may no n°er tarry in this weary conflict!

On the Value of Suffering.

(Words of the Eternal Wisdom to Blessed Henry Suso.)

In the eyes of the world suffering is contemptible, but in My eyes it is of an infinite dignity. Suffering extinguishes My wrath, gains My favor and friendship, and makes man dear and acceptable to Me.

Suffering is a hidden good which no man knows how to appreciate; and though a man were to ask for it on bended knees during a hundred years, yet he would not deserve to obtain it.

Suffering takes all that is earthly out of a man.

Suffering detaches a man from this world and wins My everlasting friendship. Believe Me, if a man only knew how profitable suffering is, he would assuredly receive it as a most precious gift from the hands of God.

Suffering preserves the soul in humility and teaches it patience; it is the guardian of purity and wins the crown of everlasting bliss. Suffering is a wholesome drink and a herb of salvation, beyond all those of paradise.   It chastens the body, which is doomed to corruption, but it gives vigor to the soul, which is far more noble and is to live forever.   Behold, the soul is nourished by suffering as the fair rose by the sweet May-dew.

Suffering is the rod of love and the paternal chastisement of My elect. Suffering draws and forces man to God even in spite of his will. Rather would I create suffering out of nothing than leave My friends without it; for in suffering virtue is proved, man ennobled, his fellow man incited to better deeds, and God is glorified.

To suffer with patience is more excellent than to raise the dead to life and perform other miracles.   It makes man a companion of the martyrs, it clothes him with a purple garment.   In suffering the soul is crowned with a garland of red roses and bears the green palm as a sceptre; in heaven she sings a new canticle, which the angelic hosts can never sing, because they have never tasted suffering. In a word, sufferers are styled miserable in this world, but I call them blessed, for they are My elect.

CHAPTER II.

Exhortation for a Worthy Reception of the Last Sacraments.

If it be a good work to console and assist the sick in their troubles, it is of far greater importance to help them to die a good death ; this indeed may be considered as the greatest act of charity, because it opens, as it were, the gates of heaven to them. If we succeed in saving a sick man from everlasting ruin by enabling him to receive the sacraments worthily, we perform the noblest work of Christianity; we fulfil the office of a guardian angel and become co-operators in the great work of redemption.

"Those who attend the sick," writes St. Alphonsus, "ought in the first place to try to learn *secretly* from the physician if the disease is mortal. I say secretly, for it is a most blameworthy practice for doctors to speak of the invalid's state in his presence, or on the other hand to conceal the danger and to flatter him with delusive hopes. If you have been told that the malady is dangerous, do not at once introduce the subject of confession, but first ask the sufferer how he is; then encourage him to resign himself entirely into the hands of God, to unite his sufferings with those of Jesus Christ crucified, and to offer them to God in penance for his sins. Then exhort him to place all his confidence in God, who is powerful enough to restore him to his former health. At the same time prudently point out to him the danger of his state, and make him understand that he must not give too much credit to doctors and relatives, as they are but too much inclined to hide the gravity of the illness in order to avoid frightening him. Then tell him it is advisable that he should make a good confession, now while he is conscious, as this will undoubtedly contribute to restore his bodily health, provided it be for the good of his soul."

I. THE HOLY SACRAMENT OF PENANCE.

As the eternal salvation of the sick man depends in a great measure upon his making a good confession, we think it our duty to treat this matter at full length in order to furnish the infirmarian with abundant matter for encouraging and instructing the sick. We take it for granted that the infirmarian is able, in case of necessity, to help the invalid to prepare for an ordinary confession, and we here add a few short instructions:

1. Exhortation to the sick to reconcile themselves with God by confession.

2. Refutation of objections usually brought forward by the sick against confession.

3. Necessity and facility of making a good general confession.

Exhortation to Reconcile One's Self with God.

When God sent word to the pious King Ezechias to announce his approaching death, and at the same time to bid him prepare for it, the king turned his face to the wall and wept bitterly at the remembrance of his sins, saying, " Lord, I will recount to Thee all my years, in the bitterness of my soul " (Cant.).

This is what every Christian ought to do at the beginning of his illness. He ought first to regulate his temporal affairs, then turn from this world to God, and in the bitterness of his soul think over his past life, sincerely repent of his sins, and confess them before God and His representative the priest.

It is highly important for the sick man to make a good confession at the very commencement of his illness. In the first place, in many cases it is only by this confession that the pains endured in the illness become meritorious for the sick man; for if he be in the state of mortal sin, however patiently he may bear his sufferings, he cannot expect the smallest reward for them in heaven. Secondly, in the Sacrament of Penance he obtains special grace from God to draw due profit from his illness for the salvation of his soul. Thirdly, as illness not infrequently is a punishment or even the consequence of former sins, so by a good confession the evil is destroyed at its root, and the recovery of health is rendered more probable. Fourthly, a good confession restores peace of mind to a troubled conscience. "A good conscience makes a soft pillow"; it sweetens everything and renders even what is hard light and easy to bear. Finally and above all, the advantage of an early confession is that one is not surprised by death unawares, unreconciled with God and summoned in this state to appear before the sovereign Judge.

The longer confession is put off the less easy it becomes. If it is found difficult to make a good confession at the very beginning of the illness, how much harder will it be when body and soul are worn out by the malady ! Is it reasonable to put off so important an affair to so uncertain a future?

See, my dear Christian, God has perhaps confined you to a bed of illness expressly for this end, that you may make your peace and be reconciled with Him against whom you have revolted like a rebel. Indeed, by your sinful life you have drawn upon yourself the anger and hatred of God; do not now hesitate nor fear to return, like the prodigal child, to your Father, whom you have so ungratefully abandoned. He invites you to do so by the voice of His Apostle (2 Cor. v. 20) when he says: "We beseech you, be reconciled to God." However grievous and numerous your sins may be, listen only to the merciful invitation of God by the prophet Ezechiel: "If the wicked do penance for all his sins, which he hath committed, and keep

all My commandments, and do judgment, and justice: living he shall live, and shall not die. I will
not remember all his iniquities" (Ezech. xviii.
21, 22). Mind well that He says: "*I will not remember all his iniquities*"—consequently all your
blasphemy, all your injustice, all your sacrilege,
all your impurity, all your drunkenness—in short,
all the sins that an impious man is able to commit,
will be forgiven you. Will you then not listen to
the sweet invitation of so good a God and root
vice from your heart? Therefore, as St. Paul
says : "Purge out the old leaven, and become a
new man " (1 Cor. v. 7); "Put off the old, the sinful man, and put on the new one, who lives in
holiness and justice, according to the image of
God " (Ephes. iv. 24).

However, in order to obtain this interior change,
the sinner must fulfil the condition upon which
entire pardon is promised to him. He must turn
to Jesus, his Redeemer, and do what He has ordained for this purpose. He is indeed our Intercessor, our Mediator, "the reconciliation for
our sins," as the Apostle calls Him; through the
merits of His blood, His passion and death, we obtain the pardon of our sins. He does not, however, confer this grace directly; He has appointed
priests to be His representatives, and it is to them
that the sinner must have recourse in order to obtain pardon; for it was to the priests God gave the
power *in His place* and in His name to forgive sins
when He said: "Receive ye the Holy Ghost;
whose sins you shall forgive, they are forgiven

them: and whose sins you shall retain, they are retained " (John xx. 22, 23).

When St. Paul, who had offended God by many grievous sins, was about to be cured of both his bodily and spiritual blindness, God directed him to Ananias, who was appointed to assist him in this important affair. The same happens to you, my dear Christian. On account of the weak and miserable state of your soul it would be too difficult for you alone to search through the long catalogue of your sins to find out all the wounds of your soul and duly to reveal them to the priest. Therefore send for an Ananias, a pastor, that he may assist you, that he may cure your wounds, which otherwise would lead your soul to everlasting death. With his assistance it will be easy for you to obtain the cure of your wounded soul; in the name of God he will pardon you, the grace of God will be bestowed upon you, and the angels in heaven will rejoice over your conversion more than over ninety-nine just men who need not penance.

Example.

In a city of the United States there lived a famous doctor, an upright and honorable man, but unhappily an indifferent Christian. Having been taken seriously ill, no one dared to advise him to send for a priest. Now it happened that exactly at this time *Bishop Cheverus* was staying in the city, and hearing of the condition of the sick man he went to see him without being invited. Having exhorted him with tender affection to reconcile himself with God, he so far prevailed upon the invalid that he asked the bishop to hear his confession. When this was done the sick man could not restrain his joy, and he thanked the bishop with the deepest emotion. He had been sad and uneasy before, but now he was perfectly calm and tranquil, and he ceased not until his death to thank and praise God for the happiness of his conversion.

2. *Refutation of Objections against Confession Usually Brought Forward by the Sick.*

1. Confession would excite me too much. This is the thought and speech not only of the sick man himself who up to this time has led an unchristian life and is afraid of confession, but also unhappily that of the relatives and friends of the patient, who are often foolish enough to shrink from speaking to him of confession, for fear of frightening him. Some of them go so far as to ask the priest on his sick-call not to speak of the patient's receiving the sacraments; he is too weak now, they say; he must be taken care of; confession would excite him too much and aggravate his state. The reply to this is that if the exertion of making a good confession would in reality shorten his life for the space of a few hours or even days, this objection is not worth any consideration if by this means eternal life and eternal bliss are secured. But this apprehension, as a rule, is an

imaginary one, since the sick man whose conscience is in order is always calmer in mind, so that even his health is benefited by his confession. The prudent confessor knows quite well that the Church does not demand from those who are seriously ill so complete an accusation as from those who are in good health; he can therefore quiet the sick man, as well as his friends, with the assurance that the confession will not take more than a few minutes, as he will only ask the most important questions. Has not the priest, before he gives absolution, sometimes to content himself with a few scanty words, sometimes even with mere signs on the part of the sick, especially when speaking is a great difficulty to them? Nay, it may even happen that he must content himself with the assurance of the persons in attendance that the sick man before losing his consciousness asked for a confessor.

Examples.

The venerable Brother *John Grande,* who had nursed thousands of sick people with the tenderest affection, frequently said that the medicine given to the sick produces a wholesome effect on the body only when the soul has been previously cured by the heavenly Physician, and reconciled with God by means of a good confession. Therefore he always insisted that every patient when he entered the hospital should first go to confession and receive holy communion.

Tissot, the celebrated Protestant physician, frequently expressed his admiration of the effects of the sacraments, in illustration of which he several times related the following example: " I had been trying every remedy in behalf of a young lady at Lausanne who was dangerously ill, but without success, and I began to entertain doubts of her recovery. The invalid, noticing this, gave herself up to excessive grief which bordered on despair. Being aware that this agitation and anxiety would only hasten the lady's death, I, contrary to my usual practice, sent for a priest. He came, consoled her, heard her confession, gave her the last sacraments, and immediately the sick lady regained her composure. On the following day I found her pulse almost regular, the fever abated, and after some time she was completely restored to health."

2. I am not yet seriously ill; later, should I grow worse, I will make my confession.

" By means of illness," says Pope Gregory, " God knocks at the heart of man, that he may open it to Him." If you open your heart to Him, you may expect Our Lord's coming with confidence. Death then will have lost its terrors for you. Therefore the saints, although constantly living in the grace of God, never failed, when ill, to purify their souls still more by the Sacrament of Penance. So the holy Bishop Wolfgang, when on a journey, being attacked by a fever, desired at once to be brought to a neighboring church, where in sight of the altar he made his confession with great humility, shedding abundant tears. Now, if the saints in the time of sickness were so anxious to purify their souls from every stain of sin, how much greater reason have we to do so ! We are poor, miserable sinners, who have done little good, but much evil. Our Saviour assures us that no one knows the hour of His coming, and that death comes like a thief in the night. Illness, therefore, is a token of His favor, a messenger sent, as it were, to admonish us : Be ready ; prepare the wedding garment, that is to say, sanctifying grace, which is necessary for entering heaven, and which is given to you in the Sacrament of Penance.

"Later on," you say, "when I am worse, I will confess." But what if death were to come suddenly, as it has happened to so many ? When you suffer from bodily illness you at once seek for help; but now that the necessary remedies for curing your soul are offered to you, you say : "To-morrow; later; not now." Is not this very imprudent, very dangerous, since the Holy Ghost threatens those who delay? "Delay not to be converted to the Lord, and defer it not from day to day. For His wrath shall come on a sudden, and in the time of vengeance He will destroy thee" (Ecclus. v. 8, 9).

"Later," you say, "when I am worse, I will receive the sacraments." Foolish man ! so then you will not look into your conscience, nor reconcile yourself with God, until you are given to understand that you have arrived at the end of your life, on the brink of the grave? Will you then be able to perform this important business better and with more facility than now, while you are yet tolerably strong and in possession of your mental powers ? The worthy reception of the sacraments, especially the making of a good confession, is a highly important matter, on which eternal happiness depends and which requires a due disposition of the soul and a serious preparation. But what sort of a confession will it be when your memory is completely debilitated and confused, your mind depressed by violent pain, your thoughts wandering? If even now you can hardly say one " Our Father " with devotion, how will you be able later to search your conscience well, to accuse yourself sincerely of so many sins, and above all to make an act of heartfelt contrition and a firm purpose never more to offend God? Do not, therefore, listen to the voice of the devil, who whispers in your ear: " There is no danger; you will not die yet; others, too, have had the same illness and yet have recovered." With these words, " You will not die," the old serpent in paradise plunged our first parents into ruin, and in like manner Satan whispers in the ear of many a sick man the same deceitful words: " You will not die; you will not die so soon," in order that he may postpone his confession, die vithout the sacraments, and so lose his soul.

Example.

A man of noble birth, but very immoral in his life, writes *Venerable Bede* in his " History of the

Church of England," was visited by his king in his illness, and urgently admonished by him to reconcile himself with God by a good confession. The sick man, however, would not consent, because he fancied that his friends would laugh him to scorn, as having, through fear of death, let himself be persuaded to confess. At length he complied so far with the urgent request of the king as to promise to confess when he was better, because then he would be able to make a better confession. After this the king repeated his visit several times, exhorting him still more urgently not to put off his confession any longer. At length he told him quite decidedly he must absolutely make his confession now, as death was already close at hand and consequently his soul was exposed to the imminent danger of being lost. Thereupon the dying man replied: " It is now too late, for I know for certain that I am damned"; and so saying, he expired.

3. Confession is a thing too difficult for me; it is many years since I confessed at all or made a bad confession; therefore I am too much ashamed.

Why so ? Are you afraid of the priest ? are you ashamed to confess your sins to him? Remember the confessor is a man, and a man as weak and sinful as yourself. St. John Chrysostom says that God has entrusted the tribunal of penance, not to an archangel, nor to an angel, but to a man, so that the priest, remembering his own weakness and sin, may show kindness to the sinner, and that the sinner himself may be encouraged to make a sincere avowal of his sins. Does not the priest each day at holy Mass thrice strike his breast, accusing himself before all the assistants of being a poor sinner ? and must he not like every other Catholic confess his sins? Why, then, should you be ashamed and afraid? The confessor, it is true, is a judge—not a judge who condemns, but one who absolves. He is that father who does not reject his prodigal son on his return home, but who receives him with joy. He is a physician—not one who cuts and burns, but, like the charitable Samaritan, one who pours the wine and oil of consolation into the wounded soul.

" Yes, that is all true," you may say; " but what will the confessor think if I confess to him so many and such grievous sins, or reveal to him those I have concealed these many, many years ? " The priest will rejoice at your humble and candid accusation and your return to God; and the greater your sins are, the greater will be his joy. He praises the mercy of God, who has borne with you so long and so patiently; he deems himself happy in being able to snatch from the clutch of Satan and to open the gates of paradise to a soul who for so many years has walked on the road to perdition. Why, then, should you be ashamed to accuse yourself of those sins which weigh so heavily on you in order to be freed from this heavy burden?

The Apostle Paul and St. Augustine have in their writings made known their sins to the whole world; why, then, should you be ashamed to confess your sins in secret to a priest? If you do not confess them now, they will on the Day of Judgment publicly be revealed to all men, angels, and saints, in presence of the thrice-holy God, to your own great confusion and your eternal damnation.

Example.

A woman who was married to an impious man had not been to confession for seventeen years, and besides this all her previous confessions had been sacrilegious. After having committed many grievous sins, she went so far as to kill her two little boys, who were unbaptized. In 1870 a mission was given in the church of St. Alphonsus in Rome. The poor woman happened to pass by the church, and, without really knowing why, she entered, and approached a priest who was hearing confessions. Upon his asking her whether she wanted to make her confession, she replied that she did not know herself why she had come there. Then the confessor with kind but earnest words invited her to perform a three days' devotion to Our Lady of Perpetual Succor, whose picture was venerated in that church. "Alas ! " replied the woman, sighing deeply, " I am lost if this heavenly Mother does not assist me. And how shall I be able to confess my countless sins ? " She followed the advice of the priest, began a three days' devotion, and before it was ended she had already commenced her general confession. When completely reconciled with God, the happy penitent was filled with such consolation that she could never cease pouring out her thanks to her heavenly

Mother, who had given her such powerful help. She also gave leave to the confessor to publish everywhere the great grace she had received from Our Lady of Perpetual Succor.

4. I am a respectable man; I have committed neither homicide nor theft; I have wronged no one. What, then, have I to confess ?

The Pharisees also did not commit external faults which would have branded them with infamy in the eyes of the world; and yet they were so guilty in the eyes of God that our divine Saviour, who had compassion on the greatest sinners, compared them even to whited sepulchres, which inside are full of dead men's bones and of all filthiness. They did not, it is true, commit homicide, but their hearts were filled with envy, anger, and hatred; they were not guilty of theft, but interiorly they were full of avarice, covetousness, and the desire of earthly things. They could not indeed be accused of open adultery, but our blessed Saviour declared to them that every one who only looked at a woman with lustful eyes had already committed adultery within his heart. If any one, after what has been said above, boasts of being guiltless, let him lay his hand on his heart and ask himself in all earnestness and sincerity: What is the state of my soul with respect to such sins as are known to God alone? What is my honesty in my occupation and in business? Is there no secret injustice? What is my temperance, what is my chastity in thoughts and desires? "If we say," writes St. John, "that we have no sin, we deceive ourselves, and the truth is not in us" (1 John i. 8). Those, however, who put forward the above-mentioned objection are usually aware themselves that it is only a mere pretence, in order to escape being obliged to go to confession; they know but too well that they have sins, and, it may be, many and heavy sins, on their consciences. Often enough they only try to cloak their want of faith by these excuses. With all the arguments of reason and faith there is no convincing such persons; therefore, instead of arguing with them, we must pray for them and try to induce them to pray themselves, especially to our blessed Lady, the refuge of sinners, as only a miracle of divine grace is able to open their eyes.

Example.

At Nocera, a small town in the kingdom of Naples, where St. Alphonsus had spent many years and where he died, there lived a very aged man. His life, it is true, had not been a bad one, but he never approached the sacraments. In April, 1881, having completed his eighty-fifth year, general debility confined him almost constantly to his bed. His pious daughter, earnestly appealing to his conscience, exhorted him to send for a priest and to confess. This request excited the man to great anger. "Confess?" said he, "what do I need to confess? I am an upright man; I have not wronged any one through all my life." The good daughter knew not what to answer, but, full of anxiety for her father's salvation, she went and told her confessor all that had happened. He encouraged her, saying: " Give this medal of Our Lady of Perpetual Succor to your father; tell him that I send it to him, asking him to wear it and to say three Hail Marys and one Gloria every day." The old man took the medal, hung it around his neck, and said the desired prayers daily. After the lapse of a fortnight, he called his daughter to his side one morning and said: " My child, I wish to make my confession. I have spent the whole night thinking over it, and longing for the morning to carry out my intention." The daughter was so amazed that she could hardly believe his words. When she prepared to go and call the priest, the old man would not allow her to do so, insisting upon going himself to the church, which was near to his house. Here he made his confession and agreed with the priest that he would return the next morning to receive holy communion. But during the night he felt so weak that he sent for the priest to bring him the holy Viaticum. His contrition was so great that he said aloud he had confessed only once before in his whole life, and that even this confession had been invalid, because through shame he had concealed one sin. He asked pardon from his daughter and every one present; then, kissing the crucifix, he died so peacefully that there is **no** room to fear for his eternal happiness.

General Confession.

A general confession is one in which the sinner accuses himself sincerely and contritely of all those sins which he has committed, either from his childhood, or since his first mortal sin, or from the time when he made a bad confession or one the validity of which he has reason to doubt.

The greatest benefit of a general confession is shown especially at the hour of death. Who would not wish to make a sincere and contrite general confession when he is about to appear before the tribunal of God ? What must be the consolation of a dying man who has regulated the affairs of his conscience before his last illness !

For Whom is a General Confession Necessary ?

1. For those who wilfully concealed a mortal sin in confession or an essential circumstance which they well knew ought to have been confessed.

2. For those who, having been grossly negligent in the examination of their consciences, have exposed themselves to the danger of not confessing mortal sins.

3. For those who in confession have made use of vague or equivocal terms, so that the confessor might not recognize the grievousness of their sins.

4. For those who have confessed merely through habit or constraint, without true sorrow for their sins and without a firm purpose of amendment.

5. For those who for a long space of time have been addicted to some sinful habit, such as intemperance in drinking, impurity, etc., without making a proper use of the means of amendment pointed out to them by their confessor.

6. For those who, in spite of their confessions, for a certain space of time have lived in an immediate occasion of sin, which they could but would not avoid.

7. For those who, in spite of their confessions, have continued to live in great enmity, without being reconciled with their neighbor or being sincerely determined to do so.

8. For those who have confessed without the sincere determination of restoring their neighbor's property or reputation.

All those were unworthy of absolution; and if they received it, it was null before God. They are therefore, under pain of everlasting damnation, obliged to make a general confession to date from the time when they first made an invalid confession.

How to Make a General Confession Easily.

Many people are frightened at the mere words " general confession," because they fancy it to be exceedingly difficult. But this is an error. With a good will and the help of a confessor it is by no means so difficult, provided you observe the following rules:

1. Seek a good and prudent confessor, and

pray to God that he may help you and by his questions render your confession easy.

2. As you are not required in a general confession to accuse yourself of venial sins, examine your conscience only on mortal sins. Especially consider against which commandments you have chiefly sinned.

3. If you have committed a sin for a long time, that is to say, if you have contracted a habit of this sin, and if you cannot remember the exact number of the sins committed, think at what age you contracted this habit, and how often you have committed the same sin in a day, a week, or a month, etc.; also try to remember whether this habit continued or whether and for how long a time it was interrupted. Then reveal it to the confessor to the best of your knowledge. For instance: " I was addicted to intemperance in drinking from my twentieth to my fortieth year about three times each month. I sinned against the holy virtue with an unmarried person during five years, nearly three times every week. During that time I made a journey and thus I did not commit that sin for six months. During that same time I consented to impure desires about two or three times a day." Or, for example: " From about my twelfth year until the present time, that is, my thirtieth year, I was in the habit of cursing and swearing, as a rule, several times a day."

4. Confess as certain what you know to be certain, and as doubtful what you know to be doubtful.

5. Let your accusation begin with that sin which causes you the greatest anxiety, for instance, with sins against chastity, with theft, and such like, if you have been guilty of them.

6. If at various times you changed your state in life—if, for instance, you formerly lived single, then married, and at last you were a widow or widower—first examine how often you sinned in the one and then how often in the other state against the same commandment.

7. It is rather inconvenient to accuse yourself in particular of all the sins committed against all the commandments in one state of life and then begin again with another state. It is better to take one commandment and go with it over all your life according to its various states and conditions.

8. It is not necessary for you to write down your confession, nor is it advisable, on account of the danger of its being found and read by others.

9. Refrain from all useless details and mention only the necessary circumstances, in decent and modest words.

10. If your confessor himself asks you any question concerning your sins, answer candidly, and then add what he may not have asked you and which nevertheless weighs upon your conscience. Be sure God does not ask you more than you are able to do, and that thus you can make a general confession without very great trouble, if you examine your conscience as mentioned above.

Example.

A French officer who, as it frequently happens among soldiers, had led a most frivolous life and burdened his conscience with a great many sins, one day when on a journey came to a place where the celebrated *Father Brydaine* was giving a mission. Impelled by curiosity to hear this great missioner, he entered the church, where the reverend father just then was speaking about the great advantages of a good general confession. This touched the old soldier's heart to the quick; he resolved at once to confess the sins he had committed from his very childhood, and he did so, shedding many tears. After his general confession, the inward peace and happiness he felt was so great that he was unable to conceal it any longer; he followed Father Brydaine into the sacristy, and there, in the presence of several priests, avowed how happy he had now become. " Gentlemen," said he, " never before have I experienced the happiness that I now enjoy, being again reconciled with God; I am firmly convinced that the King of France cannot be happier than I am, the heavy burden of my sins being lifted from my heart."

II. THE HOLY VIATICUM.

If the sick man is able to receive holy communion, tell him that the moment is not far off when

Our Lord will call him hence; he should therefore prepare for his last journey. As the passage from this life into the next is of course very painful and bitter, our divine Saviour vouchsafes to come to him by means of the holy Viaticum, in order to be his companion and support in this journey to heaven. Remind him that this is perhaps his last communion; and although Our Lord may possibly dispose otherwise, he should all the same prepare himself as if he were to receive his Saviour for the last time.

On the day when the sick man receives holy communion, bestow particular care on cleanliness and fresh air; it is well also to have perfumes ready to make use of in case of necessity.

Let the invalid's bed be covered with a clean linen cloth, or a white covering especially arranged for this purpose. Sometimes it will be necessary to raise the invalid's pillow, to allow the priest to give holy communion with greater facility.

After he has received holy communion continue to stay for some time with the sick man, to prevent him from falling asleep or expectorating too soon. Exhort him to render thanks to Our Saviour, who has deigned to visit him, and then leave him alone or, if necessary, help him to say his prayers.

The prophet Elias, being persecuted by the impious Queen Jezabel, fled into the desert to save his life. Having taken with him neither food nor drink, he sank down at the end of the first day's journey weary and heart-broken, imploring God to let him die. From the sleep into which he had fallen he was awakened by an angel, who, touching him, said: "Arise and eat of the bread which is hidden here under the ashes, for you have yet a long way to go" (3 Kings xix. 5, 6). Elias arose, ate of the bread, and gained such an increase of strength that for forty days and forty nights he walked on steadily and unweariedly to Mount Horeb, where he lived in intimate converse with God.

This angelic bread is considered by the Church as a type of that heavenly bread which we receive in holy communion, and especially as a type of the holy Viaticum. As the prophet Elias, lying worn out on the ground, was in danger of losing his life, so in like manner the sick man is in continual danger of being carried off by death. Like to the prophet, who had a long journey before him and was in need of a heavenly restorative in order to arrive at Mount Horeb, so also the sick man has the prospect of a long journey before him, for which he also wants invigorating food. This heavenly restorative is brought to him by the priest of God when he comes to his bed of pain, presenting holy communion to him, saying: "Receive, brother [or sister], the Viaticum of Our Lord Jesus Christ, that He may preserve thee from the malignant enemy and bring thee to life everlasting. Amen."

This heavenly bread is indeed the mightiest weapon against every kind of temptation with which Satan attacks those who are dangerously ill and near their end. If the mere name of Jesus, pronounced with devotion, puts the devil to flight, what will Jesus Christ Himself do when He comes to visit the heart of the sick man? What has a sick man who has thus become a living temple of the thrice-holy God to fear? How can the spirit of darkness injure him in whose soul the God of hosts has taken up His abode ? Indeed the holy Viaticum is truly that table of which David says that God has prepared it for us against our oppressors and persecutors.

What a consolation for the sick man, that the same God who soon will be his Judge now visits him as his loving Redeemer, and provides him with the means of mitigating his sentence and reconciling himself to God, giving him His merits, His blood, and His wounds in order to expiate all his offences ! Then what has the sick man still to fear? Death? Oh, no; for " he who eateth this bread," says our divine Saviour, " shall live forever." Therefore this heavenly food is called by the holy fathers a sign of predestination, a pledge of future glory, the germ and seed of immortality. St. John Chrysostom even assures us that as soon as one of the faithful has received the holy Viaticum the holy angels surround the bed of the sick man, and do not leave it until he has breathed his last.

How necessary this heavenly Viaticum is to poor sick people, and how much at the same time our divine Saviour yearns to visit and strengthen His faithful servants in this manner, God has manifested at various times by bestowing the holy Viaticum in a miraculous manner on some of His friends. Here are some

Examples.

Three times in one night the holy Bishop Honoratus was awakened from sleep and summoned to rise quickly and bring holy communion to *St. Ambrose,* who was lying dangerously ill.

When *St. Stanislaus Kostka* lay seriously ill and in danger of death at Vienna, in the house of an ill-disposed Protestant, he had not the least prospect of receiving the holy Viaticum, because his landlord would under no condition allow a Catholic priest to enter the house, and both his private tutor and his elder brother opposed his ardent wish. In this critical position he had recourse to his patroness St. Barbara, imploring her with many tears not to let him die without the holy Viaticum. Suddenly he said to a friend who was standing at his side: " Kneel down, kneel down! Behold St. Barbara, coming with two angels and bringing me holy communion ! " Then the holy young man himself knelt down, saying thrice: " Lord, I am not worthy ! " opened his mouth, and received his Saviour with the greatest humility and fervor.

Although *St. Juliana Falconieri* bore the pains of her last and protracted illness with joyful courage, she nevertheless frequently complained that on account of the nature of her illness, which prevented her retaining any food, she was deprived of the happiness of receiving the holy Viaticum. In this sad condition she asked the priest at least to deposit the consecrated Host on her breast, since she was not allowed to receive it. The priest granted her request, and lo! the very same instant the sacred Host disappeared, and Juliana soon after with joyful countenance expired. After her death the print of the Host appeared on her left side near the heart, as a sign that Our Saviour had really entered her heart.

III. EXTREME UNCTION.

When the sick man has received the holy Viaticum, prepare him for Extreme Unction by telling him that the reception of the holy Viaticum seems to have rendered him more tranquil and content. To increase his happiness he should prepare for the Sacrament of Extreme Unction, instituted by Christ, our heavenly Physician, to cancel our sins entirely and to strengthen us against the attacks of our enemies; and moreover that this sacrament has the power to restore health, provided it be conducive to our salvation.

Be careful to wash the eyes, ears, mouth, hands, and feet of the invalid, and so arrange the bed at the lower end that the covering may be easily and modestly raised when the priest has to anoint the feet.

Near the bed put a white-covered table; place

on it a crucifix and two candles, a holy-water font, some palm, a rochet, a violet stole and ritual, a plate with five or six pieces of cotton-wool or flax, and another with crumbs of bread or a little salt; also a basin of water and a towel for washing and drying the priest's hands. The cotton when used, as well as the salt and water employed for cleaning the fingers, are thrown into the fire, to prevent the holy oil from being profaned.

This sacrament is styled " Extreme [last] Unction " because it is the last of the various anointings with consecrated oil which the Catholic receives in the sacraments, viz., in Baptism, Confirmation, and Holy Orders. Our divine Saviour in His boundless love has taken care to provide that in every important circumstance of our lives His holy sacraments should be in readiness to enable us to draw the necessary graces from them, in order to attain our last end happily. Now, our last illness is a circumstance of great importance, as we are about to pass out of this life into the other; the dangers of our salvation are then singularly great, because the spirit of darkness redoubles his attacks, which on the other hand we are more than ever weak and helpless to resist, the body being racked with pain and the soul being in anguish on account of the sins committed and the judgment in view. Therefore our merciful Saviour has made provision for this by instituting the Sacrament of Extreme Unction for the sick. This sacrament, by means of the anointing with holy oil and the prayers of the priest, confers the grace of God on the sick for the good of the soul and also frequently for that of the body.

According to the teaching of the Church, *sanctifying grace is increased* within the soul by means of this sacrament. The sick man will perhaps after a brief delay be called hence into the other world; there the greater will be his bliss, the higher he stood here in the love and friendship of God. In order, then, to make him attain a higher degree of love and heavenly beatitude, God, by means of Extreme Unction, increases sanctifying grace within his soul. Another of its effects is that it effaces *venial sins* and even those mortal sins which the sick man can no longer confess. The priest while anointing the sick man asks God to forgive him the sins he has committed by his sight, his hearing, etc. The sins remitted through Extreme Unction are, first of all, venial sins. This sacrament according to its essence is a medicine of the soul; now, as medicine is given only to the sick and not to the dead, therefore Extreme Unction is in reality not instituted for those who are spiritually dead, but only for such as possess the life of the soul and consequently have only venial sins on their consciences. It may, however, occur that even *mortal sins* are remitted by means of Extreme Unction. It not infrequently happens that the sick man is no longer able to confess, because he has lost the use of speech, of hearing, or even his whole consciousness. Now, if there are mortal sins on his conscience, of which he repents at least imperfectly, they are remitted to him by means of this holy sacrament. Thus God in His infinite mercy has made provision also for these poor sinners, and many a sick man can by the help of Extreme Unction be snatched from eternal ruin, into which he would have fallen without it. Extreme Unction, however, obtains not only the pardon of unremitted sins, but it also destroys the remains of remitted sins. Among these are numbered the temporal punishments of sins which are at least partially remitted by Extreme Unction, according to the contrite and penitent disposition of the sick man. By these *remains,* however, must be chiefly understood the irregular inclinations of the heart, the weakness of the will, the dislike and indolence for good, in short all the imperfections which remain in our soul after its sins are forgiven. If a person has been cured of an illness, typhoid fever, for instance, he does not find himself at once as well and strong as he was before; he continues for some length of time to be weak and faint; he can do but little work, and must be on his guard not to have a relapse. These are the remains of the illness. The same is the case with sin. If a person has lived in sin for a long time, for instance in anger, or enmity, or impurity, and has returned to God by a good confession, still many an evil consequence of those sins remains in his soul; his will continues to be inclined to sin; he must be on his guard not to consent to temptation again; he finds little taste in prayer, is often ready to give way to discouragement, etc. These remains of sin may harass the

sick man and be accompanied by great dangers.
Then God in His mercy hastens to his assistance
by means of Extreme Unction. The grace con-
ferred by this sacrament subdues the bad inclinations, strengthens the will against temptations,
restores joy in serving God, and the soul is cured
from the remaining effects of its illness.

With this is connected another effect of Extreme Unction: *it strengthens the soul in suffering
and temptation, especially in the agony of death.*
What severe sufferings are not infrequently endured by a sick man ! To lie for weeks or months
on a sick-bed, to be racked at the same time with
violent pains, cares, and anxieties—this is no trifling thing to encounter. In order not to yield
to impatience in such a state, but to bear it willingly for the love of God, grace and strength are
required. How often will Satan make use of all
his wiles to tempt a sick man to impatience, murmurings, and complaints ! Another he surrounds
by the enticing visions of former sins to make him
yield to sinful desires. To a third he shows all
the sins of his life in the most glaring light, all
the harm he has done, all the scandal he has given,
etc., and whispers in his ear. " You have sinned
too much, too long, too heavily; there is no more
hope for you." How is the poor invalid, wearied
in body and soul, to overcome all these temptations ? Our divine Saviour in His most benign
mercy has prepared a remedy by means of which
He will support, console, and strengthen us. In
the Council of Trent holy Church declares that

" the Sacrament of Extreme Unction relieves and strengthens the soul of the sick man, inspiring him with great confidence in the divine mercy, so that, elevated by it, he is better able to bear with the troubles and hardships of illness." Consequently the effect of this sacrament is that the sick or dying man tranquilly submits to the will of God, looking forward to his end with confident hope. The Sacrament of Extreme Unction gives strength in a special manner to overcome the temptations of the evil one, to fight the good fight, and to persevere in the grace of God to the end. This efficacy of grace is symbolized by the oil with which the sick man is anointed. As the combatants of old anointed their bodies with oil to render their limbs supple and strong for the fight, so in like manner the dying Christian is spiritually anointed, and armed with the weapon of the Holy Ghost, in order to fight the last combat successfully, and to triumph over the enemies of his salvation.

Last of all, Extreme Unction frequently brings about *alleviation in illness,* and even *recovery* if it be conducive to salvation. Alleviation in illness is an effect of Extreme Unction which, as experience teaches, is not of occasional but of frequent occurrence. After Extreme Unction most of the sick feel greatly relieved; their pains are diminished, they breathe more freely, and they often say: " Indeed, now I feel well; throughout my illness I have not had such a good day." This effect, though supernatural in its origin, may be explained in part also in a natural way.   If a person has received the holy anointing with proper dispositions, interior peace soon follows in its train; the thought: "I am reconciled to God, I may hope to go to heaven," fills the soul with joy and consolation; this necessarily tells in a beneficial way upon the body, alleviates illness, and soothes pain.   Sometimes Extreme Unction brings about *perfect recovery.*   Even nowadays it happens that people who have received this sacrament in good time, and with a lively faith and confidence, obtain by it their restoration to health, without their being conscious of this grace.   Moreover, the holy Council of Trent declares that "this sacrament sometimes confers bodily health, if it be conducive to the salvation of the soul."   The sick man therefore may ask God to cure him by means of Extreme Unction, on condition, however, that it be for his salvation.   In other respects the violence of the illness is greatly reduced by the interior peace derived from the sacraments, so that medical assistance is more successful in its administration.

Examples.

St. Gebhard, Bishop of Constance, in his final illness longed for the last sacraments; and when those around him suggested that his case was not yet so serious as he imagined, he replied: "What is of paramount importance must not be delayed until we lose all our faculties and are unable to taste all the consolations which flow from the sacraments. Does not the sick man need consolation and strength? and where can he more surely find them than in the devout reception of the sacraments ? " After having received the last rites of the Church with great fervor, he joyfully exclaimed: " Now, come what may, I am united with my Saviour. If He is with me, who can be against me ? "

St. Bernard relates a miracle wrought by *St. Malachy,* Archbishop of Armagh in Ireland, from which we can see the wonderful effect of Extreme Unction as regards the body. Near the monastery of Bangor in Ireland there lived a woman who, feeling the approach of death, sent for St. Malachy. The saint came, exhorted and consoled her, and offered to give her Extreme Unction. Her friends, however, having represented to him that it would be better to put it off until the following day, he let himself be persuaded, blessed the sick woman, and returned to his cell. But when evening came the poor woman died; and when the saint heard the loud weeping and lamentation he came running to the place, and found her really dead. Conscience-stricken, with uplifted hands, he accused himself as guilty for having let the poor creature die without Extreme Unction. He at once began to pray, and continued to do so all the night. At break of day the poor woman opened her eyes and returned to life. St. Malachy without delay gave her Extreme Unction. Being restored to health, the good woman spent the rest of her days in penance, and at last she died a holy death.

St. Eleazar, of the Third Order of St. Francis, who had led a life more like that of an angel than a man, and had preserved chastity even in the married state, fell into the agony of death. His face, till then calm and serene, was suddenly disfigured, and he was heard to exclaim: " My God, how terrible is the power of Satan ! " He received Extreme Unction, and behold ! soon after his countenance once more regained its composure, and he reassured his terrified attendants, saying: " By the grace of God I have overcome ! "

IV. THE LAST EXPEDIENT (PERFECT CONTRITION).

To die without the sacraments, and without the assistance of a priest, is indeed very hard for a Catholic, and is regarded as an evil the averting of which we ask of God when we pray: " From an unprovided death deliver us, O Lord." But the decrees of God are inscrutable, and every one must be ready at any given hour to appear before the sovereign Judge. What God does is done well, and He knows what is best for every individual man. If, however, through some unforeseen accident or other circumstance, death sets in so quickly that no priest can be called to the dying man to give him the sacraments, we must not therefore lose courage and think everything is lost, but lift up our hearts to God, without whose will not a hair falls from our heads. God's mercy is wonderful and infinitely great for those who turn to Him with humility, contrition, and confidence. He never yet rejected a repentant soul truly desirous of salvation, and left it without the necessary succor in order to bring it to everlasting salvation.

If, as faith teaches us, even those who without their own fault live outside the true Church but observe the commandments of God are saved, how much more may the faithful children of holy Church hope to arrive at everlasting salvation if they do all in their power to obtain from God the forgiveness of their sins and the graces necessary for a holy death !

Now it is a dogma of the holy Catholic Church that a person even without the Sacrament of Penance can infallibly obtain pardon for all sins, even the greatest, by making an act of perfect contrition, together with a desire of receiving the Sacrament of Penance, which cannot now be received. It is therefore of great importance to know in what perfect contrition consists, and how the act is to be made. We cannot avoid treating this subject at some length.

As we know, contrition is a sorrow of the soul for sins committed, and a sincere detestation of them, combined with the purpose of never again offending God. Sin has its seat in the heart and will, and therefore also the heart must be touched with repentance, and the will, which loved sin, must hate and detest it. Where there is no repentance it is impossible for God to pardon sin, for, being a holy God, He must hate sin, and cannot love a man who continues to love sin. This repentance must extend at least to all mortal sins without exception. If any one were to exclude a single mortal sin from his repentance, God could not pardon him a single sin, because one cannot be pardoned without the other, and because by a single mortal sin we incur the whole hatred of God. It is easy to understand that God grants pardon to the sinner only when he repents of his transgressions for the sake of God; that is to say, from supernatural motives, from motives inspired by faith. A merely natural motive—for instance, because through sin one has incurred dishonor, loss of fortune or of health—is not sufficient for obtaining pardon of one's sins. Contrition which proceeds from supernatural motives may either be perfect or imperfect.

Contrition is *imperfect* when we hate and detest our sins from motives which have to do with our own eternal happiness or misery, such as the loss of heaven, the punishment of hell. Such imperfect contrition, springing from fear or hope, etc., but which yet bears in itself some beginning of the love of God, suffices to obtain the forgiveness of sins by means of the Sacrament of Penance. Without this sacrament, however, the forgiveness of mortal sins can be obtained *only by perfect contrition*, together with the will to confess. Contrition is perfect or imperfect according to the motive which makes a person hate and detest sin. Perfect contrition does not take the divine punishments for its motive; really and essentially it springs from the perfect love of God, for which reason it is also styled perfect repentance, or contrition of love. The fear of hell and the hope of heaven need not be excluded from perfect contrition; only they must, as it were, step into the background; that is to say, they must not constitute the chief motive of the contrition. He who truly loves God longs indeed for heaven, but chiefly to be there united with God, the Sovereign Good; he fears hell, but chiefly because he would there be separated from God. From the magnitude of the punishment which God inflicts upon sin, the soul recognizes the enormity of the offence committed against God. The real motive of contrition in such a soul, consequently, is the love of God, to which the fear of the divine punishments has, it is true, given the impulse.

The love of God which springs from gratitude is sufficient to obtain the pardon of sins even without the Sacrament of Penance, and consequently everlasting felicity. Truly thankful love, namely, that love which does not regard so much the gifts and benefits, but much more God, the Giver, Himself, and loves Him above all things on account of His infinite goodness, is already a perfect love; therefore also the contrition springing from it is perfect contrition. Truly thankful love gives rise in the soul to an exceedingly great sorrow for having offended so good a God, as also a hatred and detestation of sin, and a firm resolution to do and to suffer anything rather than offend that good God by mortal sin. Now, as perfect contrition, according to the teaching of the Church, reconciles us to God, it follows that it remits all mortal sins, as well as the eternal punishment due to sin. Perfect contrition makes every sinner a child of God and heir of heaven; not only the contrite Catholic, but all men, even those who without their fault find themselves outside the pale of the Catholic Church, provided they are so disposed as to be ready to receive the sacrament in case they recognize this obligation. Therefore, also, one must not despair of the salvation of even the greatest sinner, especially when he is on the point of departing from this life. The grace of God does not take long to change the heart of the sinner. It sometimes lights up and softens the soul with lightning-like rapidity. Even a heretic, a Jew, or a heathen may therefore obtain everlasting felicity if on his death-bed he turns to God, makes an act of perfect contrition, and at the same time wishes to do what, with the grace of God, he deems to be necessary for salvation. God wills that all men should be saved. He offers to all men the help of His grace; he only who rejects it is lost forever.

An act of contrition does not by any means depend on the words or the formula, but on the disposition of the heart. Contrition must be in the heart, in the will; words are only the means to express this interior disposition. If, therefore, we here give a few formulas for making an act of perfect contrition, we must before all be certain that the words come from the heart.

Act of Contrition. (*Long Formula.**)

O infinitely merciful God, graciously look on me, a poor and miserable sinner. With an humble and contrite heart I confess before Thee: " Father, I am no longer worthy to be called Thy child." Who will give a fountain of tears to my eyes, that I may weep over my ingratitude and malice towards Thee, O Sovereign Good ! Incline and soften, O God, my heart to true repentance and detestation of my sinful life. Yes, I am sorry, and repent with all my heart for having so often and so grievously offended Thee, my heavenly Father, my kind and loving God, especially by those sins. [Here recall your mortal sins.] For these and all the sins of my whole life, for those I know and those I do not know, I am sorry from my inmost soul, not only on account of the punishments I deserve for them in this and still more in the other world, but especially for the love of Thee, because I have been so disloyal towards Thee, my most loving Creator, the best of Fathers, and my supreme Benefactor, and have repaid Thee with so much ingratitude. Above all I am sorry for my sins because thereby I have offended Thee, who art the Sovereign Good, who art infinitely good, infinitely holy, and art worthy to receive infinite love and honor from all Thy creatures.

O my God and my Supreme Good, now I love

---

* To be used by all who believe in God and life eternal.

Thee with all my heart; and because I love Thee I hate and detest all my sins, and entreat Thee for the sake of Thy infinite goodness and mercy to forgive me. With Thy assistance I firmly purpose to do everything Thou requirest of me, especially to amend my life and rather die than ever again to offend Thee, my God, by mortal sin. Amen.

Act of Perfect Contrition.

(To be used by Catholics only.*)

O my God, Lord of heaven and of earth, Thou hast loved me from all eternity; Thou hast loved me so much as to deliver up Thy only-begotten Son unto death. How should I not love Thee with all my heart in return? Yes, I love Thee more than all the things of this world, because Thou art infinitely good and in Thyself worthy of infinite love. Now, because I love Thee with all my heart I repent of, hate, and detest most sincerely all the sins, and especially all the mortal sins, by which I have ever offended Thee, my most amiable God. Forgive me, O most merciful Jesus! I firmly purpose [to confess my sins] to amend my life, and for nothing in the world wilfully to offend Thee again. Jesus, give me the grace to keep my resolution. Amen.

* For Protestants it may be used by omitting the words in brackets, " to confess my sins."

Abridged Act of Perfect Contrition.

I love Thee, O my God, with all my heart, and I am sorry above all things for having offended Thee, O Infinite Goodness ! Oh, purify me by the merits of the passion of Thy divine Son Jesus !

Examples.

In the reign of Queen Elizabeth *Lord Stourton* was unfortunate enough to give up his religion. When he came to die, he could not find a priest to hear his confession and reconcile him to God and to holy Church. So, in order to obtain pardon of his many grievous sins, he had no other means left than to make an act of perfect contrition. Not content with this, he caused his whole family to assemble around his death-bed, and protested in their presence his heartfelt repentance for his sinful life, and his sincere desire to die as a member of the Catholic Church; whereupon he asked them to publish this protestation. As Lord Stourton had died repentant, Father Cornelius, S.J., who afterwards was martyred for the faith, said Mass for him in the chapel of the house. After the consecration the persons who were present saw on the side wall of the chapel the reflection of a burning fire, while the priest saw an immense sea of fire, and in the midst of it the deceased nobleman, who with tears and painful groans accused himself of his misdeeds, especially of his having been accessory to the condemnation of the innocent Queen Mary Stuart. When Mass was over the priest addressed the persons assembled, and declared to them that the deceased nobleman had found grace with God and saved his soul, but that he had much to suffer in purgatory.

In the life of *Sister Mary Dionysia* of the Visitation Order we read that Our Lord one day showed her the soul of a mighty prince in purgatory. He had been killed in a duel, but had received the grace to make an act of perfect contrition before he breathed his last. Our Lord then ordered the Sister to offer a great many prayers and mortifications for the repose of his soul, which she faithfully performed throughout the remainder of her life. This prince, in the fear of death, had, as it were, instinctively invoked God's help, obtained a moment's consciousness, and with it the grace of repentance, by which he secured everlasting life.

CHAPTER III.

Method of Willingly Accepting Death.

(From the writings of St. Alphonsus.)

The Venerable Lewis Blosius assures us that he who in health makes an act of perfect conformity to the will of God will be preserved not only from hell, but also from purgatory, though he might have committed all imaginable sins. The reason is that by accepting death with perfect resignation the soul obtains a merit equal to that of the holy martyrs, who willingly sacrificed their lives for Christ. "Yes," says St. Thomas, "it is truly to be a martyr when a person suffers death for practising an act of virtue." From this we must infer that a man acquires the merit of martyrdom not only when he gives his life for the faith by the hand of the executioner, but also when he accepts death to render himself conformable to the will of God and to please Him. This is the highest act of virtue a man can perform, making an entire offering of himself to the divine Love. As regards the *kind of death*, we must be convinced that the death which God has decreed for us is the one which is best for us. Therefore, as often as we think of death we should say: "Lord, let me die as it pleases Thee, only let me obtain eternal salvation." Also, with regard to the *time* of our death we must be entirely resigned to the will of God. This earth is nothing more than a prison in which we must suffer and in which we are every moment liable to lose God. Therefore the Royal Psalmist exclaimed: " Lead my soul out of the prison ! " Penetrated by the same sentiment, St. Teresa longed for death, and on hearing the clock strike rejoiced that one hour more of her life had passed away, and with it also one hour of the danger of losing God. According to St. John of Avila, every one who is only moderately well prepared for death should wish for it, as we all live in great danger of forfeiting the grace of God. By a happy death we obtain the certainty that we shall never lose the grace of God. How could there be anything more precious, more desirable than this certainty? Therefore, also, the saints yearned unceasingly for their heavenly home, precisely because they were inflamed with the love of God. David lamented his long exile: " Woe is me, that my sojourning is prolonged ! " Only the hope of everlasting felicity could console him. " I shall be satisfied when Thy glory shall be made manifest " (Ps. xvi. 15). St. Paul had no greater desire than to depart from this life in order to be with Christ. " The good for which I hope," said St. Francis of Assisi, " is so great that every suffering is delightful to me." All these manifestations of *yearning desire* are so many acts of perfect love. St. Thomas teaches that the highest degree of **love** which a soul can attain in this life consists in the ardent desire of heaven, there to be united with God and to possess Him.

The greatest pain of the poor souls in purgatory consists in their longing for the possession of God, and this pain is especially the lot of those souls who on earth had little desire of heaven. Cardinal Bellarmin even thinks that there is in purgatory a place (he calls it the honorable prison) where the souls suffer no pain of the senses, but are tortured by the privation of the Beatific Vision. St. Gregory, St. Vincent Ferrer, St. Bridget, and the Venerable Bede quote several examples of such punishments which were inflicted, not on account of sins committed, but on account of a deficiency of desire for heaven. Indeed, many souls aim at perfection, without longing to quit the earth and to arrive at union with God. Now, as eternal life is an infinitely precious gift, purchased for us by the death of Jesus Christ, those souls later on have to suffer punishment on account of the little desire they had for it during life.

Example.

A pious countryman having in his illness manifested a desire to be favored with the blessing of *St. Francis of Sales,* the kind-hearted bishop readily complied with his request. " Your lordship," the sick man immediately said, " shall I die of this illness ? " " I have," said the saint, " seen many persons, whose cases were far worse than

yours, return to health. Confide in God, who is the
Master of life and death." " But do you think I
shall die ? " " A doctor would be able to answer
that question better than I," replied the saint.
" The best thing for you would be not to trouble
yourself about it—to deliver yourself into the
hands of God, who will do what is best for you."
" My lord," replied the good peasant, " I do not
ask you this because I fear to die, but because I
fear *not* to die. It is hard to think of a recovery."
" There is no doubt," said St. Francis, " that you
have heavy cares in your position, since life is such
a burden to you." " By no means, my lord; I have
everything here that I desire; but in the sermons
I have heard, the life to come and the joys of
heaven are so much extolled that this world seems
to me a prison." And then the good man, from
the fulness of his heart, spoke so beautifully
about paradise that the holy bishop shed tears of
joy and admired the Spirit of God, who had so
well instructed this unlettered man.   Then the
pious invalid made an act of resignation to God's
will as to life or death, and, a few hours later,
gently fell asleep in the Lord, after having received the sacraments of the Church.

GENERAL ABSOLUTION

in the hour of death is by no means, as some erro-
neously believe, a last absolution or acquittal of all
the sins of the whole life, but only a remission of all

the remaining temporal punishments due for sin; that is to say, a plenary indulgence in the hour of death, otherwise simply styled " indulgence at the hour of death." In her maternal love the Church once more opens her treasures of grace to her children before they go out of this world, granting them this plenary indulgence, that so they may be enabled, by means of the infinite merits of Jesus Christ and of His saints, to make up for their deficiencies, to make atonement to the divine justice, and without delay to enter into everlasting joy. Now, what has the sick man to do in order to gain this indulgence?

1. He must have the will or *intention* to gain the indulgence. There is no doubt that every dying Catholic has this desire; wherefore the indulgence, according to the express declaration of the Church, can be given to those who are left without consciousness, and even to madmen.

2. He must be in a *state of grace,* which is the case with those who have already worthily received the sacraments. Those who cannot confess and communicate must at least make an act of perfect contrition if they are in a state of mortal sin. To this end the following act of perfect contrition may be read to them: " O my God, I am heartily sorry for having so often and so grievously offended Thee, who art my Creator, my Redeemer and Saviour, who hast loved me with infinite love. O sovereign and most loving God, how could I be so ungrateful and malicious as to offend Thee so much ? "

3. He must, either orally, or, if this is not possible, at least in his heart, *invoke the name of Jesus.* This may be done by saying, for instance: "Jesus, help me! Jesus, be merciful to me! Jesus, pardon me my sins!"

4. He must *willingly accept* the sufferings of illness and even death from the hand of God as an atonement for his sins. Let the sick man be particularly reminded of this point as one of the chief conditions for gaining the indulgence. With many of the sick this will have to be done with extreme care, and this sometimes more out of regard for their surrounding friends than for themselves. It is often easiest to do this when one is alone with the sick man, by suggestions such as these: "Willingly will I suffer, O Jesus! Willingly will I die, making Thee atonement, O God, for my many sins by my suffering and my death."

Remark.—The same conditions are required if a person possesses some object which has the power of an indulgence at the hour of death, such as a cross, a rosary, or a medal, or is a member of a Confraternity to which a plenary indulgence is granted at the hour of death. Those indulgences can be gained, as well as the general absolution, without the assistance of a priest, only the possessor must carry these objects about with him, or at least have them near—for instance, hanging against the wall—and in sight of them perform the devotions prescribed.

CHAPTER IV.

Assistance in Temptations.

" THE life of man here on earth," says holy Job,
" is a continual warfare." In days of health, but
especially in days of sickness, new temptations and
new combats are continually succeeding each
other. Therefore we must be ever ready to meet
with temptations, and not disquiet ourselves, however great their violence and frequent their return may be. We must console ourselves with the
consideration that in all our tribulations God as-
sists us with His grace and will not allow us to be
tempted above our strength, as St. Paul says :
" God is faithful, who will not suffer you to be
tempted above that which you are able; but will
make also with temptation issue, that you may be
able to bear it " (1 Cor. x. 13).

The holy Council of Trent in particular teaches
that the enemy of the human race exerts all his
powers and artifices to effect our ruin and if possible to rob us of confidence in God's mercy at no
other time so much as when he sees that our life is
drawing near its end. Prayer, above all, is a most
effectual antidote against all sorts of temptations.
With the sick man this has to consist chiefly of

short ejaculations, especially of frequent invocation of the most holy names of Jesus and Mary. " In the name of Jesus every knee should bow, of those that are in heaven, on earth, and under the earth," writes the Apostle Paul (Phil. ii. 10); and " Whosoever shall call upon the name of the Lord shall be saved " (Acts of the Apostles ii. 21). " Strike thy enemies in the name of Jesus," says St. John Climachus, " for there is no more powerful weapon either in heaven or on earth."

As long as you are able to speak, have this name constantly on your lips; when you can do so no longer, invoke it in your heart. Holy Church has granted an indulgence of twenty-five days to those who devoutly pronounce this holy name, and a plenary indulgence at the hour of death provided they invoke it at least in their heart.

Also the holy name of Mary is terrible to the demons, since it is the name of the holy Mother of God, who crushed the serpent's head. "As soon as the evil spirits hear the name of Mary," says St. Bridget, " they leave the soul." " There is no army on earth so much in dread of the enemy as the powers of hell are of the name of Mary and of the assistance thereby obtained," says St. Bonaventure. The servant of God, Sertorius Caputo, therefore exhorts those who assist the dying to recall to them frequently the holy name of Mary; " for," he says, " if the dying invoke this name in the hour of death it is enough to drive away all their enemies and to console them in all their anguish." So, then, make use of these holy names as a firm buckler; call out with heart and lips, "Jesus! Mary!" and the tempter will take to flight. Imitate the saints, who made frequent use of these weapons.

But among the many temptations there are a few against which a sick man must be provided in a special manner. These are:

I. TEMPTATIONS AGAINST FAITH.

Faith is the foundation of our salvation, the anchor of our hope, and the best consolation in life and death. This is what the wicked enemy well knows; therefore he strives above all to shake our faith; he tries also to deprive the sick man of his faith in God's wise providence, making him believe that He neither knows anything about him nor cares for him. Moreover, he disturbs the sick man with various doubts about certain truths of religion, and endeavors to tempt him to reason indiscreetly on the mysteries of our holy religion.

Let us hear what St. Alphonsus writes concerning faith and the temptations against it: "Our Lord God wills that we should have our understanding, in order to recognize with certainty that it is He who has spoken, but not in order to comprehend what He presents to us to be believed. Reason takes us, as it were, by the hand, and leads us into the sanctuary of faith, but then remains itself standing at the threshold. As soon as we are convinced that the doctrines which we are asked to receive faithfully really come from God, we must submit our understanding and, on the word of God, admit as truth whatever is presented to us to be believed, although we are unable to comprehend it. The mysteries of faith are not at variance with our reason, but they exceed its power of comprehension. Therefore we must not enter into subtle reasonings about them in order to penetrate them, lest our fate be that of those haughty minds who, attempting to get an insight into these mysteries, are deserted by their weak understandings, and entangle themselves in a multitude of difficulties from which they hardly succeed in disengaging themselves."

" Faith," says St. Augustine, " is not a matter for the proud, but for the humble " (Serm. 115, n. 2). To believe is not difficult for him who is truly humble.

If, therefore, any one is tempted by the devil in matters of faith, let him by no means enter upon the difficulties which the enemy brings forward, but let him make an act of faith and protest before God that he is ready to give his life in testimony of the holy faith. St. Francis of Sales was once, when ill, greatly troubled with doubts in matters of faith concerning the holy Eucharist. But he in no way entered into a parley with the devil, defeating him simply by the invocation of the name of Jesus. In temptations of this kind we must therefore in all humility surrender our understanding, submit to the teachings of the Church, and beat the devil with his own weapons, protesting: "I am ready to give my life a thousand times for the holy faith." If we act thus, we shall find a source of merit in what the devil has designed to be harmful to us.

Quite in the same sense, and entering more into particulars, the Venerable Father Martin of Cochem says: "Suppose the thought arose in your mind whether until now you had lived in the true faith, or whether there are three persons in one God, or whether Jesus Christ can be present in the Most Holy Sacrament, and so on. You should not dwell upon this thought, much less reason about it, whether it is so or not; for if you were to do so, surely the enemy would deceive you or plunge you into some error. Therefore do not stop at such thoughts, do not reflect upon them, much less dispute with the enemy; on the contrary, give up these thoughts, think of something else, and act as if you did not even notice them. But if nevertheless they worry you, and will not let you have any peace, say in your heart or with your lips: 'Jesus! Mary!' 'Jesus, guard me!' 'Jesus, preserve me in the true faith!' If you are still able, say the Apostles' Creed as attentively as you can, or say in your heart: 'I believe what the Catholic Church believes, and in this holy Catholic faith do I desire to live and die.'"

Examples.

When *Blessed Columba of Riéti*, of the Third Order of St. Dominic, lay dying, God permitted

that her innocent and much-favored soul should
be violently tempted by the devil in various ways,
especially with regard to faith; her face even reflected the grief and anguish of her soul.   But
she in no wise intended to give way to the suggestions and sophisms of the wicked one, and said
imploringly: " Lord Jesus, help me ! " repeated
the Apostles' Creed, and continually asked the
assisting priest, as well as her Sisters, to do the
same.   After half an hour's struggle against the
spirit of darkness and unceasing invocation of
the holy name of Jesus, the enemy was at length
obliged to desist, and no longer disquieted her.

Frederick Ozanam, the well-known and illustri-
ous French author (1853) writes the following in
his last will: " To-day, as I finish my fortieth year,
and am suffering in body but sound in mind, I
have written my last will in a few words, resolving
to express it more fully when I am stronger. . . .
I abandon my soul to Jesus Christ, my Saviour,
with fear on account of my sins, but with confidence in the infinite mercy of God.   I die within
the pale of the Roman Catholic Apostolic Church.
I have got acquainted with the scepticism of the
present century, but my whole life has brought
home to me this conviction, that there is no rest
for the spirit and the heart but in the faith of the
Church and under her authority.   If I set any
value on my long studies, it is because they confer on me the right earnestly to entreat all those
whom I love faithfully to adhere to a religion in
which I have found light and peace.   My last re-

quest to my family, my wife, my child, my brothers and brothers-in-law, as well as to all their descendants, is to persevere in the faith in spite of the humiliations, scandals, and apostasy of which they will be witnesses. . . ."

II. TEMPTATIONS AGAINST HOPE.

On account of their sins, and through fear of the divine judgment, the sick frequently fall into very low spirits, and the wily enemy avails himself of this to plunge them into despair. A person, then, renders herself guilty of the sin of despair if she thinks only of God's strict justice without confiding in His infinite mercy, if she is only in fear of God without hoping in Him, if she, therefore, like Cain the fratricide, thinks in her heart, " My sins are too great and too numerous for God to forgive them." In time of illness man ponders over his former life; he remembers many sins he has committed, and recognizes many a thing to be a sin which he formerly did not heed at all. This remembrance and bitter acknowledgment should stir him up to a more heartfelt repentance, and should urge him to confess his sins and to make what reparation he can for what has been done. But the enemy who formerly deluded him with the idea that the sin was not so grievous, and that later on he could repent of it and change, because God is so infinitely merciful, does exactly the contrary now. He suggests the thought that it is now too late; that he has offended God too much and too long to be able to be converted and to hope for forgiveness from God. But the infallible Church, supported by the word of God, teaches that every one, even the very greatest sinner, can procure the pardon of his sins as long as he lives, and up to the last moment can obtain grace and pardon from God. This we see from the good thief on the cross, who in his last moments was converted, and heard the consoling words: " This day thou shalt be with Me in paradise " (Luke xxiii. 43).

Therefore St. Cyprian says: " Repentance never comes too late, if only it is sincere." And in another place he writes: " Neither the grievousness of sins nor the shortness of time excludes pardon, if only there is true repentance and genuine conversion of the bad will." Our divine Saviour also said, one day, to St. Catharine of Sienna: " Those sinners who mistrust My mercy, and at the end of life give themselves up to despair, offend Me more by this one single sin than by all the sins which they have committed before."

If the sick man is disquieted and tempted to despair by the remembrance of his sins, let him reanimate his confidence in God by the following considerations, which are mostly extracted from the writings of St. Alphonsus.

The first motive of our hope is the *boundless mercy of God*, for God is called, and in truth is, a Father of mercies. He desires, much more than we do ourselves, to make us happy forever. He loves us more than a mother does her dearly loved child. He goes in search of us like a shepherd for his lost sheep. He is ever ready to pardon the repentant sinner. He testifies on oath that He willeth not the death of the sinner, that is to say, his eternal ruin: "As I live, saith the Lord God, I desire not the death of the wicked, but that the wicked turn from his way, and live" (Ezech. xxxiii. 11). He assures us that if the sinner detests his iniquities He will no longer think of them: "If the wicked do penance, I will not remember all his iniquities" (Ezech. xviii. 21).

Who, then, could doubt God's mercy after such declarations from Eternal Truth? One single sigh of contrition from the heart of the sinner suffices to obtain pardon for even the greatest sinner, if he has the sincere desire to amend, and to confess his sins as well as he can.

"Yes," one perhaps may think, "but I am not an ordinary sinner; I am more criminal than others; my sins are more numerous than the hairs on my head. For me there is neither help nor hope nor pardon." What? Will you put bounds to the mercy of God ? I tell you, God's mercy is infinitely great, greater than the greatest sin. No, not I, God Himself tells you this: "If your sins be as scarlet, they shall be made as white as snow: and if they be red as crimson, they shall be white as wool" (Isa. i. 18). Yes, as soon as a contrite heart implores His pardon, He is at once ready to grant it; in one instant He cleanses the soul which for years had been scarlet with the blood of sin. No sooner had the publican in the

Gospel said, with a contrite heart, " Lord, be merciful to me, a poor sinner," than he was justified
before God.   Hardly had David acknowledged
his sin and owned it, saying, " I have sinned,"
than Nathan, by the order of God, announced to
him forgiveness, saying: " The Lord has taken
away thy sin."

Example.

Blessed Clement Hofbauer one day called on a
man sick unto death, who had not been to his duty
for twenty-two years, and who even on his death-
bed refused to receive the sacraments. As he answered the exhortations of the servant of God only
with abuse and slander, and bade him withdraw,
Father Hofbauer retired a little, but remained at
the door, contemplating him while he recited the
Rosary. " What do you want here ? " cried the sick
man. "Go, and leave me in peace." "As your end
is so near," answered Blessed Clement, " I shall
not go away. I have often been witness of a happy
death; to-day I want to see how one who will be
damned will die." These words startled the sick
man, and completely changed him.   Full of
shame, contrition, and fear, he called the servant
of God to his bedside, and said to him in an entirely different tone: "Father, can you forgive me
for all the abuse I have heaped on you? " And
as Father Hofbauer answered, " Everything has
already been forgiven," the sick man continued:
" But will God also forgive my sins? " The ser-

vant of God answered: "God is infinitely merciful; make an act of contrition for your sins and God will forgive all." The sick man now made a contrite confession, pressed the crucifix which Father Hofbauer gave him to his heart, and died in the peace of the Lord. Father Hofbauer himself narrated this conversion as a plain proof of the extraordinary and infinite mercy of God.

A second motive of confidence is the *Passion of Jesus Christ*, who protests that He has come into the world only to save sinners and to make them happy forever: "I have not come to call the just, but sinners" (Matt. ix. 13). It is true, indeed, that we have to render a strict account to God for all our sins, but who will be our judge? Let us be of good heart; "the Father hath given all judgment to the Son" (John v. 22).

It is Our Saviour Himself to whom the Father has assigned the judgment. Therefore St. Paul encourages us, saying: "Who will judge us? Jesus Christ, who died, yes, who also maketh intercession for us" (Rom. viii. 34). We shall be judged by our divine Saviour, who, to avoid condemning us, delivered Himself up to death for us, and who, not satisfied with this, continually makes intercession for us with His Father in heaven. "What, then, do you fear, sinner?" says St. Thomas of Villanova, "if only you detest your sins? How could He condemn you, who died to avoid doing so?" If only you become repentant, how could He cast you off? He came down from heaven to seek you, when you fled from Him. St. Chrysostom says that each of the many wounds of Jesus Christ is a mouth which is continually speaking and imploring God's pardon for our sins. At the fatal moment when we committed sin God wrote the sentence of our eternal damnation. But what did Jesus Christ do ? He took, as the Apostle says, this sentence of condemnation, obliterated it with His blood, and fixed it to His cross, that we might never look at it without seeing also the cross on which He annulled it, that so we might have the hope of pardon and eternal salvation. "Blotting out the handwriting of the decree that was against us. . . . He hath taken the same out of the way, fastening it to the cross" (Coloss. ii. 14). "Let us go therefore with confidence to the throne of grace: that we may obtain mercy in seasonable aid" (Heb. iv. 16). The cross is the throne of grace on which Jesus Christ is placed in order to bestow His graces and mercies on all those who put their trust in Him. The merits of Jesus Christ have unlocked for us the treasury of God, since they entitle us to whatever graces we can wish for. St. Leo remarks that the advantages which Jesus Christ gained for us through His death are far greater than the injury which the devil has done us through sin. St. Paul also teaches that the donation which God has made to us by redemption is far greater than the loss we have suffered through sin: "But not as the offence, so also the gift; . . . and where sin abounded, grace did more abound" (Rom. v. 15, 20).

St. Eleazar, after having led an extremely pure life, was violently tempted at the hour of death; but he by no means lost courage, saying to those around him: " The efforts of hell at this moment are very great, but Jesus Christ, through the merits of His Passion, deprives them of all power."

Examples.

In the life of *St. Frances of Rome* we find the following event: One day, the saint having been sent to assist a young man who was dying in a hospital in Rome, she heard a shriek in an adjoining ward.   Hastening thither, she beheld a young woman in danger of dying in despair.   Enlightened by God, Frances beheld her dangerous state. She was an infanticide, but her crime was wholly unknown to others.   As she approached her end, she had not the courage to own it in confession, and consequently was in imminent danger of being lost.   Then the saint, by the most touching care, endeavored to win her confidence and to move her to make a contrite confession.   At first the sick woman paid no attention to the saint, who never ceased to point out to her the extreme danger of her soul, showing her how ready God was to pardon her numberless sins, and how one single tear of repentance, together with the blood of Christ and a good confession, would blot out her guilt and win for her everlasting happiness.   Then at length the sinner's heart gave way.   She burst into tears, asked for a confessor, accused herself

of her crime with heartfelt contrition, and received the last sacraments. But the saint never
left her, lovingly exhorting her to unite her sufferings with those of Jesus Christ, and to receive them as a penance for her sins. " If Satan
wants to tempt your faith," said she, " do not enter
into a dispute with him; tell him plainly that you
believe what the holy Catholic Church teaches,
and keep firmly to it. If he wants to rob you of
your confidence by whispering into your ear that
you have not made your confession well, answer:
' I hope that, through the mercy of God, my confession was good. Grievously ill as I am, I could
not clearly remember the past; if I have forgotten
something, I repent of it from pure love of God,
who is infinitely good and amiable.' " The sick
woman listened to the words of the saint with
every sign of contrition, and a few hours later expired peacefully and resignedly in the arms of
Jesus.

St. Bernard when thinking of his sinfulness was
frequently visited by fear and despondency. A
pious and confident look directed heavenward was
enough to restore his cheerfulness. " Do not despair, my soul," said he to encourage himself, " do
not despair; for since Jesus Christ ascended to
heaven, we have there a Mediator, an Intercessor, a
Redeemer. I know this well. I acknowledge that,
on account of my sins, I do not deserve heaven,
but Jesus Christ, my Saviour, does possess it, and
He possesses it for a twofold reason: first, because
He is the Son of God; and secondly, because He

purchased it with His own blood. The former
is enough for Him, but as for the latter, He leaves
it to me. By virtue of these titles I have a claim
to heaven, and I do hope to obtain it, through the
love of Jesus Christ, my Redeemer and Intercessor,
and the mercy of my Heavenly Father."

A third motive of confidence consists in *the
promises of God.* Holy Scripture offers us the
most powerful motives for unshaken hope in God,
as it were, on every one of its pages. There we
read that God promises everlasting salvation and
the assistance necessary for obtaining it to every
one who prays and hopes: " Whatsoever you ask,
when ye pray, believe that you shall receive: and
they shall come unto you " (Mark xi. 24); " Every
one who asketh receiveth " (Matt. vii. 8); " The
Lord is a protector to all those who hope in Him "
(Ps. xvii. 31); " My children, behold the genera-
tions of men: and know ye that no one hath hoped
in the Lord, and hath been confounded " (Ecclus.
ii. 11); " None of them that wait on Thee, shall
be confounded " (Ps. xxiv. 3); " In Thee, O Lord,
I have hoped, let me never be put to confusion "
(Ps. lxx. 1); " Because he hoped in Me I will deliver him and I will glorify him " (Ps. xc. 14, 15);
" Amen, amen, I say to you: If you ask the Father
anything in My name, He will give it you " (John
xvi. 23). These, as well as other innumerable
promises, are addressed to all men without exception, not only to the just, but also to sinners. It
is therefore sufficient to ask God with an upright
heart for the graces necessary to salvation, and He

will assuredly grant them: " The Lord is good to
the soul that seeketh Him " (Lament. iii. 25).

Example.

Baron Moser, living in Vienna, suffered for a
long time from a disease of the chest, which, however, he did not consider to be dangerous, and therefore refused to receive the sacraments. The baron-
ess, his pious wife, entreated Blessed Father Hofbauer to prevail upon her sick husband to receive
them without delay. The servant of God came
and said to him: " Baron, make your confession
and be assured that you will go to heaven."
Greatly astonished at this assurance, the baron replied: " What do you say, Father Hofbauer ? Is
that really true? " " Quite certain," replied the
holy man. " If this be so, I will confess at once."
He did so, full of joy at the consoling assurance
given to him, and died resigned to the will of God
and in the firm hope of obtaining everlasting life.

A fourth reason for our confidence is the *intercession of the Blessed Virgin.* " Great and singular
in its kind," says St. Bonaventure, " is the privilege of Mary, that by her intercession she obtains
from her Son whatever she wills." However, of
what avail would this power be if Mary did not
take care of us? But no; as she is a more powerful intercessor with God than all the rest of the
saints, so also is she more loving and more solici-
tous for our good than all the rest. (Spec. B. V. 1,
6). She loves us because her beloved Jesus en-

trusted us to her care when just before His death He addressed her, saying: " Woman, behold thy son " (John xix. 26). She loves us because for our sakes she suffered such great sorrow, for mothers usually love those children more whose lives were purchased by a greater measure of sufferings and hardships. Now, we men are those children, for whose sake Mary underwent this excruciating suffering in consenting to sacrifice the life of her dear Son Jesus on the cross—in seeing Him die before her eyes in untold anguish in order to acquire for us the life of grace. In this very fact we behold a fresh reason why Mary loves us so much. It is because she beholds in us the price of the blood of Jesus Christ. Why, then, should she not love us tenderly, when her Son loved us to such a degree as to give His life for us? When she sees a sinner praying at her feet, she does not look at the guilt, but at the disposition with which he comes. If his intention be good, she receives him graciously, though he may have committed all possible sins; she then endeavors with great solicitude to cure all the wounds of his soul, because she is not only in name but also in reality the Mother of mercy.

As she is *our life* during our exile here on earth, so also she will be *our sweetness* at the end of our earthly pilgrimage, obtaining for us a calm and happy death.

Example.

In the revelations of *St. Bridget,* approved by the Church, we read that the Blessed Virgin Mary communicated to the saint in what special manner she had protected her son Charles at the hour of his death. " Before he gave up the ghost," said the Mother of God, " I stood near thy son, that no earthly affection might captivate him, and that he might not speak, think, or do anything displeasing to God or prejudicial to his soul. I assisted him also at the momentous hour of death, lest he might suffer too great agony and thus lose perseverance and forget God in the end. I also screened his soul from the devil and his angels, so that none of them could touch it, but as soon as it left his body I took it under my protection. The host of evil spirits who in their malice wished to torment this soul, and devour it forever, immediately took to flight."

III. TEMPTATION TO IMPATIENCE.

" The merit of crosses," says St. Francis of Sales, " does not consist in their weight, but in the manner in which we bear them. He who suffers illness with reluctance and vexation, far from diminishing his pains, rather augments them. For as all things which we do willingly and joyfully become easier, so, on the other hand, everything, even what is most easy, becomes heavy and oppressive as soon as we do it unwillingly and with reluctance." " He that is patient," says the wise Solomon, " is governed with much wisdom: but he that is impatient exalteth his folly " (Prov. xiv. 29).

Moreover, he who willingly accepts from the hand of God the pains of illness will obtain not only relief from them, but will also have less to suffer in purgatory, and receive an exceeding great reward in heaven. " Your sorrow," says our divine Saviour, " shall be turned into joy " (John xvi. 20).

But if a person bears illness with impatience she not only loses these benefits, but moreover commits many a sin, and incurs new guilt and punishment for eternity. St. Cyprian says: " What patience builds up for heaven by good works is demolished by impatience." This, however, does not mean that every manifestation of pain, or every revelation of it to others, is a sign of impatience and consequently a sin. "There is," says St. Francis of Sales, " a great difference between complaining and manifestation; you may tell what pain you suffer, but it must be done quietly, without exaggeration or murmuring. After the example of our divine Saviour, we should accept and bear with the same resignation whatever God sends us, be it agreeable or disagreeable." Being asked how she could continue to be so cheerful in her great suffering, St. Angela of Foligno answered: " Believe me, we do not know the value of suffering, for if we did we should meet it as a prize, and every one would snatch the opportunity of suffering from his neighbor." As St. Paul says: " The sufferings of this time are not worthy to be compared with the glory to come, that shall be revealed in us " (Rom. viii. 18).

The following considerations may be of use by way of exhortation to the sick man : Consider what great harm you do to yourself if you give way to impatience, if you complain of the long duration of your sickness, of the doctor, of his prescriptions, of the nursing, of your relatives, etc., or if you allow yourself even to murmur against God. You refuse to carry the cross after your Saviour, to tread in His footsteps; you are, then, only a Christian in name, since a Christian must be a follower of Christ. Moreover, as often as in your suffering you give way to impatience, fretfulness, and anger, you lose one of those pearls with which God meant to adorn your crown in heaven; but as often as for the love of Christ you overcome your impatience and your anger, you insert a new pearl in that crown. Before all things have recourse to prayer, that God may strengthen you to practise patience, for by ourselves we cannot do the least good, but we can do all things in Him who strengthens us; and He bestows strength on all who humbly and perseveringly ask Him for it, according to His promise : " Every one that asketh receiveth " (Matt. vii. 8).

Examples.

Like holy Job under the Old Law, so does *St. Lidwina*, among all the saints of the Christian

Church, shine as the most accomplished model of patience in enduring illness. She was born at Schiedam, in Holland, of wealthy parents. When she grew up, as she was endowed with singular beauty, there was no lack of suitors; but she asked God and the Blessed Virgin to change her so that no one henceforth might find any complacency in her. In the fifteenth year of her age this prayer was heard; for while she amused herself skating with other girls on Candlemas-day according to the national custom, a young friend in stumbling pulled her down, and Lidwina in her fall broke the short rib on her right side. In consequence of it internal abscesses formed which, in spite of all the remedies employed, could not be healed. For the space of three years she languished on her sick-bed, during which time she was occasionally able to get up and to be carried to church. But then began for her a bitter passion of thirty-eight years, which were spent almost entirely in bed. All the attempts to make her take invigorating food were in vain, immediate vomiting being the invariable consequence. One of the tumors gradually developed and spread throughout the whole body, causing her unspeakable pain. In three places they broke out, and thus large wounds were formed. Moreover there was hardly any illness by which Lidwina was not visited : intermittent fever, headache, toothache, dropsy, pestilential boils, and finally a most painful internal malady. She entirely lost the sight of one eye, and could see but little with the other. In the course of time a large wound opened from the brow to the chin, as though the head were split in two. Somewhat later her suffering was increased by a wound in her thigh and so great a relaxation in all her limbs that for the space of seven years she could only lie on her back, unable to move any member but her left arm. The first three years, indeed, she still longed to recover health, but her confessor having recommended her to seek solace in the wounds of Jesus Christ, meditation on the Passion of Our Saviour now became her continual occupation, and thus these constant illnesses grew more and more dear to her, as she beheld in them a means to become conformable to Him who had by suffering proved His love for her. Later on she used to say that if by means of one single Hail Mary she could recover her health she would not say it, but would let the will of God be accomplished in her. The last remnant of her strength was exhausted by a fit of vomiting which continued from morning until night. On the third day of Easter week, 1433, she sank into a swoon, from which she never awoke. Soon after her death her features were wonderfully transformed, the wound in her face closed, and she looked as youthful and blooming as if illness had never touched her.

Although afflicted by God with five very painful maladies, *St. Camillus of Lellis* bore them with so much patience and joy that he called them " special mercies of the Lord." The first ailment was an incurable wound which in his very youth had opened at the ankle-joint, and it continually tormented him for nearly forty-six years until his death. He always bore it with unshaken resignation and incomparable patience, and derived great benefit from it, convinced as he was that God had sent him this suffering in order to make him know what sick people frequently have to suffer. The second affliction was a serious rupture which he had contracted by his incessant and excessive exertions in the service of the sick, and which during thirty-one years forced him to wear a truss of tremendous pressure, which caused him unspeakable anguish.

The third illness was occasioned by three callosities under the sore foot, which were so hardened and painful that the streets became paths of thorns for him, and if at times he hobbled, it was not so much on account of the wound, as of the violent pain produced by the aggravation of these callosities. He bore this cross for twenty-five years, and it served to remind him at all times that this earth is strewn with thistles and thorns, and that he must hasten to win the unfading crown of eternal life.

The fourth evil from which he suffered was a disease of the kidneys producing a great number of calculi, which from time to time had to be removed, causing him indescribable pain.

The fifth and last illness was a constant nausea for every kind of food, so that he was seen involuntarily to shudder at even hearing it mentioned. It was probably thirty-six months that he suffered this misery with extraordinary patience, till at

length it brought him to the grave. Yet all the
time he returned thanks to God, because he learned
from it that the end of his earthly pilgrimage was
at hand, and that in this poor valley of exile he
should only yearn for the heavenly joys.

IV. TEMPTATION AGAINST CHARITY.

Many a one says: " I am good to those who
deal kindly with me; but as for ingratitude, I cannot stand that." To such our divine Saviour says
that even the heathen are thankful to those who do
them good, but that a Christian must wish and do
good even to those who hate and do evil to him.
" But I say to you: Love your enemies, do good to
them that hate you, and pray for them that perse-
cute and calumniate you " (Matt. v. 44).

If you pardon the offence done to you, you are
sure to obtain pardon from God, as He has said:
"Forgive and you shall be forgiven" (Luke vi. 37).
When St. Elizabeth of Thuringia was praying one
day for a person who had offended her, Our Lord
said to her: " Know that you have never said a
prayer more pleasing to Me than this; behold,
therefore, I forgive you all your sins." On the
other hand, Our Saviour assures us that he who
does not forgive may not hope for forgiveness from
God. " If you will not forgive men, neither will
your Father in heaven forgive you your offences "
(Matt. vi. 15). We all have offended God more or
less, and offended Him much oftener and more

grievously than others have offended us. Now, just as we wish and hope to obtain God's pardon for our sins, so also must we readily forgive our neighbor. But if you do not pardon your neighbor, God in His turn will not forgive you. To find no pardon of one's sins—what a distressing thought! And yet it is so: no pardon for you unless you have previously pardoned your enemy. You will be treated like the merciless servant in the gospel. "The lord grew angry," says Holy Scripture, "and delivered him up to the torturers." So God will punish every one who is uncharitable, both here on earth by the torments of a bad conscience, and in eternity by the torment of the worm which never dieth, and of the fire which is never quenched.

Do not follow the principles of the blind world, which considers it cowardice and shame to pardon an enemy; follow rather the example of Jesus Christ, the Infallible Wisdom, who even on the cross forgave and prayed for His cruel enemies and murderers. Far from lowering yourself by such a mode of acting, you raise yourself to a high degree of virtue and earn the approval of God. St. Stephen prayed for those who stoned him; St. James the apostle embraced his accuser before his execution; St. Ambrose caused a sum of money to be given to an assassin who had aimed at his life, and thus procured an honest living for the man; St. Louis (Louis IX., King of France) invited to his table the man who had designed to murder him. Some one, perhaps, may object to this, saying: " But these were saints; I do not possess so much moral strength." Listen to what St. Ambrose tells you in reply: " If you are deficient in strength, ask God for it, and He will give it you."

Examples.

St. John Gualbert while still a worldly-minded nobleman had the misfortune to lose his brother by the hand of an assassin. He determined to take a signal revenge, and sought for his enemy everywhere, but in vain. It happened, one Good Friday, that he met him in a narrow ravine; he was alone and unarmed, and escape was impossible. John unsheathed his sword with a gleaming eye and a heart full of rage. Then his enemy fell prostrate at his feet, and with uplifted hands implored mercy and pardon for the love of Him who on this day had on the cross pardoned His murderers. John paused a moment to reflect; a violent struggle took place in his soul; but grace conquered, and in his turn falling on his knees he embraced the guilty man and said: " Yes, for the love of Him who this day died on the cross I forgive you, that my sins may be forgiven me." Then John entered the first church he came upon, full of repentance for his sins, drew near to the cross which on this day was exposed for the veneration of the faithful, kissed it, and devoutly prayed: " O Jesus, who hath said, ' Pardon, and you shall be pardoned,' behold, for the love of Thee I have forgiven my enemy; so then, in like manner, for-

give me my many and grievous sins." And, oh
miracle ! Our Lord loosened one hand from the
cross, and bent down to embrace John as a token
that He had really pardoned his sins.

Charles III., King of Spain, before receiving
Extreme Unction was asked by the priest whether
he forgave his enemies. Upon which the sick man
gave this truly Christian and royal answer:
" Would I have waited for this momentous hour to
do so? No, I pardoned them as soon as they had
offended me."

V. TEMPTATION OF ATTACHMENT TO LIFE.

We are only pilgrims and strangers here on
earth, as Holy Scripture says; we have no perma-
nent abode here. One day we all must die; for it is
appointed unto man once to die: a few years
sooner or later makes no difference in the end, if
only we die well. With all his heart, therefore,
should a sick man thank God, whose mercy has
not let him die in the state of sin, but has given
him time and opportunity to receive the sacraments, so that, being cleansed and strengthened by
them, he may be able to pass happily unto a better
life.

Young people, especially, often find it very difficult to die at so early an age; but if you take a
right view of life, you will see that it can be called
neither long nor short. " Life," as Holy Scripture says, " is nothing but a fleeting cloud, a pass-

ing shadow, a wind hurrying along with exceeding swiftness." Even though you had attained the age of Mathusala (nearly a thousand years), still death would come too early for you. And if you continued to live seventy or eighty years more, they would soon pass away, and then, after all, you would have to die. But it is.doubtful whether you would then die well, for a long life does not make a man better. On the contrary, the longer a man lives, the more he sins, the greater is his responsibility before God and the more numerous are the punishments for sin which he has to expiate. It is not a misfortune to die early, for here on earth we are exposed to so many dangers and temptations that the longer we live the greater is the danger of being lost forever. As often, therefore, as St. Teresa heard the clock strike she rejoiced that another hour was past in which she was in danger of losing her God.

The sick man might object, saying he wished to live longer only to be able to do penance for his sins and to atone for the past by a more regular life. To this plea St. Alphonsus replied: " No penance is more pleasing to God than to accept death willingly as an atonement for sins committed; and there is no action more perfect and more pleasing to God than to die willingly, when and how it pleases Him."

Example.

A rich man one day entreated *St. John the Almoner* to pray to God for the recovery of his only son, who was ill; with this intention he also gave to the saint a sum of money, to be distributed to the poor. The holy man complied with the request; nevertheless the son died. Then the father was deeply grieved, thinking that the prayer and alms offered for his child had been in vain. The saint, noticing the dejection of the man, besought God to console him; and his prayer was heard, for one night an angel came to the distressed father with the following message: "The prayer for your son has been heard, and through it he lives in heaven, and is happy. To obtain heaven it was time for him to die; for had he lived longer he would have grown vicious and have forfeited everlasting glory."

VI. TEMPTATION OF ATTACHMENT TO EARTHLY THINGS.

Let those whose hearts cling to earth, and who therefore do not wish to die, consider that these perishable things are in reality not true but only apparent goods, which God in a thousand various ways can take from us, which at any rate we can only possess for a short time here on earth, and which do not give lasting peace to those who enjoy them; as King Solomon from personal experience confesses, saying that all the goods of this world are nothing but vanity and affliction of mind. Therefore our divine Saviour calls the rich man in the gospel a fool, because after an abundant harvest he hoped to find his happiness in these earthly goods. " Thou fool, this night do they require thy soul of thee, and whose shall those things be which thou hast provided? " (Luke xii. 20.) He who does not willingly disengage his heart from these earthly things will be separated forcibly from them by death; but then it is to be feared that together with temporal goods he will also forfeit eternal ones. Let us therefore frequently meditate on the great and beautiful things God has prepared for us in heaven; then we shall find that death does not bring us loss, but great gain, since to a Christian who dies in the state of grace it gives a thousand times more than it can take away. Therefore St. Gregory writes: " If we consider what great things are promised to us in heaven, then everything possessed on earth appears to us trifling and paltry."

If it is hard for the sick man to leave his wife, his children, or other near relatives, let him take this to heart, that a true Christian must be ready to part for God's sake with even what is dearest if He should ask the sacrifice. He who is not determined to do this must not flatter himself that he is a true disciple of Jesus Christ, as Our Saviour has said: " He that loveth father or mother more than Me is not worthy of Me " (Matt. x. 37). Moreover, let the sick man consider that now he must be intent only on securing his own salvation; and that in heaven he will be much better able to provide for his dear friends and pray for them, that they also may enjoy everlasting bliss; one day he will see them again in heaven and be united with them in unalloyed felicity throughout all eternity. Finally, the sick man should not forget that in heaven he will find far better friends than those he is now leaving behind, namely, his beloved Redeemer, the Blessed Virgin, and all the angels and saints.

Let the poor sick man who fears that after his death his family will be destitute be reassured by the reflection that God, the best of fathers, is in a special manner the protector of widows and orphans, and that He who feeds the birds of the air will provide for them; and finally that the sick man himself, when he goes to heaven, by his intercession at the throne of God can benefit them more than on earth.

Example.

Cornelius à Lapide relates the following striking event: " I once knew a very rich man, who in his last moments convoked all the inmates of his house, that they might help him to ward off the stroke of death. He caused his wife and children to appear before him, and said to them: ' Dear wife, beloved children, help me in this awful hour; have I not worked day and night for you ?' 'Alas !' they replied with tears, ' what can we now do for you, father? What can we do against so incurable an illness? Oh, would to God we could save you ! But we are not able to do so. Alas ! there is no remedy against death.' ' Ah, death !' cried the invalid, 'must I then positively die? Oh, how vain and foolish are all the endeavors of men! For you, my wife, for you, my children, have I worked in the sweat of my brow; for you have I toiled and exhausted myself; for you have I offered up my strength, my health, and my life, perhaps even lost body and soul! And for all this, such is my reward! I invoke your aid in the hour of death, and you are not able to help me! Oh, would that I had made friends for myself in heaven! In this dread moment they would have come to my assistance. Oh, how differently would I live had I the happiness to recover!' But this repentance was fruitless, this promise came too late! Death took hold of this rich man, snatched him away from all the things to which his heart was fettered, and dragged him before the tribunal of God."

CHAPTER V.

Conduct in Protracted Illness.

It frequently happens that illnesses last a long time, for months and even for years, without the sick man being able to see a prospect of perfect recovery. Some of these maladies are accompanied with acute pain; others indeed are less painful, but produce tediousness, weariness, and depression of mind. Imagine a man suffering from dropsy, or consumption, or cancer, etc.; how many sleepless nights, how many harassing days, has he to pass until death frees him from his misery! Is it, then, strange that such invalids are exposed to many grievous temptations? At one time they are tempted to impatience and disgust of life; at another time they give way to murmurs and vexation against their friends; and then, again, they are displeased with the ordinances of God, and doubt His providence and love. In such cases it is the duty of the Christian infirmarian to encourage and console these sorely tried souls with heartfelt sympathy, making use of all the arguments which reason and religion suggest to enable them to resign themselves to God's will and bear their sufferings cheerfully. They ought to take all possible care that this long illness may become for their patients a means to amend their lives, to grow in virtue, and to enrich them with merits for eternity. Patients of this sort are very frequently troubled with temptations such as: " I cannot work, and I am a burden to others; I cannot pray nor go to church; all the doctors and medicines in the world will not cure me, and I am not even allowed to complain." The answer to this kind of temptation has been given already (pp. 120, 124); only let it be observed that these unfortunate creatures really deserve especial sympathy, and even though they sometimes make their sufferings the favorite topic of conversation, this is easily understood and also pardonable. Infirmarians must with very great patience make such invalids the peculiar object of their solicitude. Above all, let them try to divert their minds in a manner corresponding to their position, their education, and their state of health, even by light reading. But then it is also a duty to occupy them with God and holy things relating to their salvation and their present state, which can best be done, first, by providing them from time to time with suitable spiritual nourishment; secondly, by endeavoring to keep them united with God in an easy and simple way; thirdly, by directing their devotion to the Passion of Our Lord, which is the best school of consolation for sufferers.

The best spiritual nourishment for the soul is to be found in the words of Holy Scripture coming from the Holy Ghost Himself, in the lives

of the saints, as also in the golden book of the
" Imitation of Christ."   Among the lives of the
saints the preference is to be given to those which
are written in a simple style, not too long and
adapted to the state of the sick man.   We append
a number of texts drawn from Holy Writ, suitable
for enkindling in the soul the virtues especially
necessary for the sick man; and also a list of chapters from the " Imitation of Christ " peculiarly
fitting for invalids.

Exercise of Various Christian Virtues, drawn from Holy Scripture.

INVOCATION OF THE DIVINE AID.

" O God, come to my assistance; O Lord, make
haste to help me " (Ps. lxix. 2).

" My soul is troubled exceedingly: but Thou, O
Lord, how long?   Turn to me, O Lord, and deliver
my soul: O, save me for Thy mercy's sake " (Ps.
vi. 4, 5).

" O Lord, my God, in Thee have I put my trust:
save me and deliver me " (Ps. vii. 2).

" O God, my God, look upon me: why hast
Thou forsaken me?   For tribulation is very near:
for there is none to help me " (Ps. xxi. 2, 12).

" My strength is dried up like a potsherd "
(Ps. xxi. 16); " for Thou art God my strength "
(Ps. xlii.).

" Thou art my helper and my deliverer: O Lord,
make no delay " (Ps. lxix. 6).

" My soul is sorrowful and refuses to be comforted " (Ps. lxxvi.). "Be Thou my comfort, O God of all comfort " (2 Cor. i.).

" I am poor and sorrowful: for the waters of affliction are come in even unto my soul. O God, attend to my soul and deliver it " (Ps. lxviii.).

ACTS OF FAITH.

" Lord, I believe in Thee: increase my faith " (Luke xvii. 5).

" Lord, I believe in Thee, the eternal Truth; and though I should die with Thee, I will not deny Thee " (Matt. xxvi. 35).

" I know that my Redeemer liveth, and in the last day I shall rise out of the earth: . . . and in my flesh I shall see my God. Whom I myself shall see, and my eyes shall behold, and not another " (Job xix. 25–27).

" Yea, Lord, I believe that Thou art Christ, the Son of the living God, who art come into this world " (John xi. 27). "Not to destroy souls, but to save " (Luke ix. 56).

" For ever, O Lord, Thy word standeth firm " (Ps. cxviii. 89).

ACTS OF HOPE.

" In Thee, O my God, I put my trust; let me not be ashamed " (Ps. xxiv. 2).

" Have mercy on me, O Father of mercies, and God of all comfort " (2 Cor. i. 3).

" Have mercy on me, O God, have mercy on me: for my soul trusteth in Thee, and in the shadow of Thy wings will I hope " (Ps. lvi. 2).

" The Lord is my light and my salvation, whom shall I fear? The Lord is the protector of my life, of whom shall I be afraid ? " (Ps. xxvi. 1.)

" For though I should walk in the midst of the shadow of death, I will fear no evils: for Thou art with me, O Lord " (Ps. xxii. 4).

" The Lord is my helper and my protector: in Him my heart confideth and I shall be helped " (Ps. xxiii.).

" We have an advocate with the Father, Jesus Christ the just; and He is the propitiation for our sins and for those of the whole world " (1 John ii. 1, 2).

" The Lord is compassionate and merciful: long suffering and plenteous in mercy " (Ps. cii. 8).

" As a father hath compassion on his children, so hath the Lord compassion on them that fear Him: for He knoweth our frame " (Ps. cii. 13, 14).

" As I live, saith the Lord God: I desire not the death of the wicked, but that the wicked turn from his way, and live " (Ezech. xxxiii. 11).

" Come to Me, all you that labor and are burdened, and I will refresh you " (Matt. xi. 28).

" Commit thy way to the Lord, and trust in Him, and He will do it. He will save you, because you have hoped in Him " (Ps. xxxvi. 5).

" He that putteth his trust in Me shall inherit the land, and shall possess **My** holy mount " (heaven) (Isa. lvii. 13).

DESIRE OF GOD AND OF HEAVEN.

" Lord, I desire to be dissolved and to be with Christ " (Phil. i. 23).

" As the hart panteth after the fountains of waters: so my soul panteth after Thee, the strong and living God " (Ps. xli. 2).

" For Thee my soul hath thirsted. . . . When shall I come and appear before the face of God ? " (Ps. xli. 3.)

" I rejoiced at the things that were said to me: We shall go into the house of the Lord " (Ps. cxxi. 1).

" Bring my soul out of prison to the heavenly home, that I may praise Thy name " (Ps. cxli. 8).

" How lovely are Thy tabernacles, O Lord of hosts: my soul longeth and fainteth for the courts of the Lord " (Ps. lxxxiii. 2, 3).

" Better is one day in Thy courts above thousands of years spent in all the possible enjoyments of this valley of tears " (Ps. lxxxiii.).

ACTS OF THE LOVE OF GOD.

" I love Thee, O Lord, my strength, my refuge, and my deliverer " (Ps. xvii. 2, 3).

" I found Him whom my soul loveth: I held Him: and I will not let Him go " (Cant. iii. 4).

" Let us love God with all our heart; because God first hath loved us " (1 John iv. 19).

" My love is Jesus crucified, who loved me and delivered Himself for me " (Galat. ii. 20).

" Who then shall separate me from the love of Christ ? " (Rom. viii. 35).

ACTS OF CONTRITION.

" O Lord, have mercy on me a poor sinner" Luke xviii.).

" Have mercy on me, O God, according to Thy great mercy; and according to the multitude of Thy tender mercies blot out my iniquity " (Ps. l. 3).

" O Lord, wash me yet more from my iniquity, and cleanse me from my sin " (Ps. l. 3).

" Father, I have sinned against heaven, and before Thee: I am not worthy to be called Thy son " (Luke xv. 2).

ACTS OF PATIENCE.

" Whom the Lord loveth, He chastiseth: and He scourgeth every son whom He receiveth " (Heb. xii. 6).

" My soul, take all that shall be brought upon thee: and in thy sorrow endure, and in thy humiliation keep patience; for gold and silver are tried in the fire, but acceptable men in the furnace of humiliation " (Ecclus. ii. 4, 5).

" God forbid that I should glory, save in the cross of Our Lord Jesus Christ " (Galat. vi. 14).

" All the sufferings of this time are not worthy to be compared with the glory to come, that shall be revealed in us " (Rom. viii. 18).

" If we suffer with Christ, we shall also be glorified with Him " (Rom. viii.).

ACTS OF RESIGNATION TO THE DIVINE WILL.

" My Father, if it be possible, let this chalice pass from Me; nevertheless not as I will, but as Thou wilt " (Matt. xxvi. 39).

" As it hath pleased the Lord, so is it done: blessed be the name of the Lord " (Job i. 21).

" Father, Thy will be done on earth as it is in heaven " (Matt. vi. 10).

" If we have received good things at the hand of God, why should we not receive evil ? " (Job ii. 10).

Chapters of the "Imitation of Christ," Adapted for the Sick.

I. TO MAINTAIN PATIENCE.

Book III. Chapter 12.—On learning patience.
"   "   "   29.—The time of tribulation.
Book II. Chapter 9.—Want of all comfort.

II. TO STRENGTHEN CONFIDENCE.

Book III. Chapter 30.—The divine assistance.
"   "   "   50.—An offering to God.
"   "   "   59.—All our hope in God.

III. ABANDONMENT TO GOD.

IV. TO PROMOTE CONTRITION AND HUMILITY.

V. TO ENKINDLE THE LOVE OF GOD.

Bk.   II. Ch.   8.—Of familiar friendship **with** Jesus.

Bk. III. Ch.   5.—Of the wonderful effect of divine love.

"   "   "   6.—Of the proof of a true lover.

"   "   "   10.—That it is sweet to despise the world and to serve God.

"   "   "   21.—That we are to rest in God above all goods and gifts.

VI. ENCOURAGEMENT BY THE EXAMPLE OF CHRIST.

Bk.   I. Ch.   1.—Of the imitation of Christ, and the contempt of the vanities of the world.

Bk. III. Ch. 18.—That temporal miseries are to be borne with equanimity, after the example of Christ.

"   "   "   56.—That we ought to deny ourselves, and imitate Christ on the cross.

Bk.   II. Ch. 11.—Of the small number of the lovers of the cross of Jesus.

"   "   "   12.—Of the royal road of the holy cross.

Bk.   I. Ch. 18.—Of the example of the holy fathers.

VII. CONSOLATION WITH A VIEW TO ETERNITY.

Bk.   I. Ch. 22.—Of the consideration of **human** misery.

VIII. THE FOUR LAST THINGS OF MAN.

To keep the sick man united with God by good thoughts, there is a simple method which consists in making use of every-day occurrences or of the objects surrounding the sick man, so as to bring them in connection with God and to deduce from them salutary reflections, pious affections, and good resolutions. The following may be serviceable on such occasions:

Various Opportunities to Remind the Sick Man of God and Holy Things.

(According to P. L. Scupoli, Theatine.)

1. After the Physician's Visit.—You do not object to any prescription given you by an earthly doctor, and you willingly take his bitter medicines, in order to recover your bodily health; show your-

self as obedient and as docile towards Jesus
Christ, the heavenly Physician, by accepting every
trial from His hand, and resigning yourself entirely to His holy will; He sends them for your
good.   An earthly doctor does not take the bitter
drugs which he prescribes for his patient, nor
does he take upon himself his patient's illness and
pains in order to cure them. But see, your
heavenly Physician bore Himself our maladies and
pains, in order to work out our salvation.   How
great is His love !

2. *After the Visit of Sympathizing Friends.*—
See how many come to visit and to console you;
but while your Saviour was hanging on the cross,
desolate and abandoned, His enemies gathered
round to insult and mock Him: on the very cross
they did not leave Him in peace.   Every one has
sympathy for you, but for Jesus His holy Mother
alone with St. John and Mary Magdalen had compassion; and the sight of His sorrowful Mother
only augmented His torments.

3. *The Sick-bed.*—It is indeed trying and painful to lie all day and night in bed, and through
exhaustion and weakness to be unable to walk.
But consider the hard bed of the cross on which
your Saviour hung in death.   When an infant
He lay on rough straw in a stable !   You at least
have a bed, but Jesus had nowhere to rest His
head.

4. When the sick man suffers from bed-sores he
does not know on which side to turn or where to
lie for rest.   Think of Jesus on the cross.   See,

He was obliged to bow His head on account of the painful crown of thorns; His holy hands and feet were fixed with nails to the cross; He was not able to move.

5. *The Night.*—It is hard if all through the night you cannot sleep. Then you count the minutes until day. But think of the poor souls in purgatory, how long they must suffer; and how easily, by a patient endurance of your illness, you can shorten or even annul the punishments of purgatory.

6. *The Night-light.*—Let the light burning so quietly at your bedside put you in mind of the altar-lamp before the Blessed Sacrament. Adore Jesus in spirit, and ask Him to enlighten you and to keep the darkness of sin far from your soul.

7. *The Clock.*—Does not its striking tell you that another hour of your life is spent, and that you are approaching your end ? Therefore avail yourself of the precious time for gathering a few more merits for eternity. Be patient, offer your pains to God; for behold, perhaps the hour is not far off when God, if you suffer for His love, will change your pains into joys.

8. *The Cock's Crow.*—St. Peter wept when he heard the cock crow. Could you not also, as often as you hear the cock crowing in the night, think of your sins, repent, bewail them, that you also may obtain forgiveness ?

9. *The Looking-glass* shows you your face with its marks of suffering. The best mirror for you is Jesus on the cross, and Our Lady of Dolors

under the cross. Often contemplate them and suffer in union with them.

10. The Rosary is a distinguishing mark of the servants of Mary; it teaches you how to love Jesus with Mary, to follow Him on the way of the cross, and to earn the unfading crown which is promised in heaven. If you cannot say the rosary, at least from time to time salute Mary with an Ave.

11. On Washing your Face and Hands.—You clean your face, my dear friend; the most lovely countenance of Jesus was sullied with the spittle of a rude soldiery! Sigh to Jesus, saying: "O my Saviour, with Thy precious blood cleanse me from all my sins!"

12. When the Sun Shines into the Sick-room.— See how the sun shines and brightens all; how it warms and vivifies everything! It is an image of Jesus Christ, whom Holy Scripture styles the Sun of justice. He is your light, your l'fe; raise your eyes, hands, and heart to Him, entreating Him to enlighten you with the rays of His grace, to enkindle the fire of His love within your heart, and to be a lamp to your feet on the way to eternity.

13. On Gazing at the Moon and Stars.—Oh, how beautiful it must be there beyond the stars, where God is enthroned in His glory, where the saints shine brighter than the stars! There, my heart, beyond the skies, you will find rest and peace!

14. At the Sight of Flowers placed near the bed.— Our Lord God has planted you as a flower in His garden, the Church; there you should blossom and fructify. After a short delay He will transplant you into the heavenly garden, where the spring is endless, and where you are to blossom forever. The flowers of this earth quickly fade and fall off. Man alike blooms and fades away after a short time. But on the day of the resurrection the just man will rise to a new life, to bloom forever in the kingdom of heaven !

Devotion to the passion of Christ was the favorite devotion of all the saints; it was the book from which they learned that science of the saints which made them friends of God; from this they drew the strength steadfastly and even joyfully to persevere amid all the trials of life. " As to me," St. Bernard writes, " from the very beginning of my conversion, when I realized my want of virtue, I provided for myself a spiritual bundle of myrrh, composed of all the sorrows and bitternesses of my Saviour, and fixed it to my breast. As long as I live its remembrance will never fade from my memory. I have found that it is wisdom to contemplate these things, and have recognized that herein alone consists perfect justice, most sublime science, riches of salvation, and abundance of merit."

You also must make for yourself a little nosegay out of the sufferings of Jesus Christ; adorn your breast with it and let it lie there; for if you have it thus continually before your eyes, and consider the sorrows of Our Saviour, you will, supported by Him, more easily endure your own sufferings.

Therefore endeavor frequently to recall to your

memory the Passion of our divine Saviour, and to compare His pains with your own; this contemplation will, with the grace of God, render your sufferings easy to bear, nay, even agreeable and pleasant.

If, for instance, you are troubled with a *violent headache*, think of the frightful pains which your Saviour suffered when crowned with thorns.

When your *teeth ache*, remember the buffets which your Saviour endured for you.

When your *hands and feet* are aching, consider the cruel nails which pierced His holy hands and feet.

When you are under the pressure of great *languor* and *weakness*, contemplate your Jesus weak unto death under the weight of the cross.

When you are tortured by interior *heat* and *thirst*, think of the torment of your thirsting Saviour on the cross, and of His plaintive cry, " I thirst ! "

If your *couch* is very hard, if your body is sore from lying so long, think how your Saviour had to rest on the hard cross, with His body all covered with wounds.

When *medicines* are very bitter and distasteful, then think of the gall and vinegar which were presented to your Saviour.

If you *cannot sleep*, remember the agony of your Saviour in the Garden of Olives and the many ill-treatments He had to endure the following night.

If you are left *without care* and *consolation*, con-

sider the abandonment of Jesus on the cross, and
also the scorn and derision He met with.

If you are sorely tried by *perspiration,* think of
the bloody sweat and agony of your Lord.

If you have no *appetite,* think of the hunger
and thirst which your Jesus frequently suffered.

Whatever sort of pain is racking you, whatever
may be the illness you endure, think that your
Saviour had suffered far more. All the tortures, pains, and sorrows of the world—your own
included—did He bear; with boundless love for
you did He endure such untold sufferings, in order to obtain for you the strength patiently to endure your sufferings through love of Him.

Clock of the Passion of Christ.

(By the Venerable F. Passerat, C.SS.R.)

AT SIX O'CLOCK (EVENING).

*Jesus, after having taken leave of His holy Mother,
goes to eat the Last Supper with His disciples.*

Admire the excess of love of Jesus Christ and
render Him thanks for His sufferings and for the
merits of which He then made us partakers, and
say to Him lovingly and devoutly:

" O my Lord Jesus Christ, blessed be the hour
in which Thou didst manifest Thy desire to enter
upon Thy passion ! *I unite all my actions and
sufferings with this adorable mystery. Through*

Thy divine merits, O Jesus, remember me at the hour of my death and be merciful unto me."

AT SEVEN O'CLOCK (EVENING).

Jesus washes His disciples' feet and institutes the Sacrament of His love.

Admire the humility with which Jesus Christ washes His disciples' feet, and the love which prompts Him to give Himself as our nourishment.

" O my Lord Jesus Christ, blessed be the hour in which Thou didst institute the Most Holy Sacrament of the Altar ! I unite all my actions and sufferings . . ." (as above).

AT EIGHT O'CLOCK (EVENING).

After the Last Supper Jesus holds His last discourse, and then goes into the Garden of Olives.

Adore the Sacred Heart of Jesus, which, quite inflamed with the love of men, now for the last time feeds His disciples with the bread of His holy doctrine.

" O my Lord Jesus Christ, blessed be the hour when Thou gavest us Thy last instructions, which, proceeding from the most tender love, were confirmed by the wonderful example of Thy sacrifice on the cross ! I unite all my actions and sufferings . . ." (as above).

AT NINE O'CLOCK (EVENING).

Jesus praying prostrate on the ground: " My Father, if it is possible, let this chalice pass from Me; nevertheless not as I will, but as Thou wilt."

Admire the perfect resignation of Thy Saviour.

" O my Lord Jesus Christ, blessed be the hour in which Thou didst with such great love accept the chalice of Thy bitter passion ! I unite all my actions and sufferings . . ." (as above).

AT TEN O'CLOCK (EVENING).

Jesus enters upon His agony and endures a bloody sweat.

Adore the Sacred Heart of Jesus as the source of eternal life.

" O my Lord Jesus Christ, blessed be the hour in which Thou wouldst be encompassed with anguish and filled with bitterness for us sinners ! I unite all my actions and sufferings . . ." (as above).

AT ELEVEN O'CLOCK (EVENING).

Jesus strengthened by an angel.

Adore our divine Saviour as the Truth which enlightens the world, and as the Life which animates it.

" O my Lord Jesus Christ, blessed be the hour in which, to console us in our weakness, Thou

wouldst deign to accept consolation from an angel ! I unite all my actions and sufferings . . ."
(as above).

AT MIDNIGHT.

Jesus betrayed by Judas and bound with cords.

Adore our divine Saviour bound with chains of love.

" O my Lord Jesus Christ, blessed be the hour in which Thou didst choose to be bound, in order to draw us to Thyself by the sweet bonds of Thy love ! I unite all my actions and sufferings . . ."
(as above).

AT ONE O'CLOCK (MORNING).

Jesus led to Annas; He receives a blow on His face, and speaks meekly to him who strikes Him.

Admire the unspeakable meekness of Jesus Christ.

" O my Lord Jesus Christ, blessed be the hour in which Thou wouldst suffer insult that we might learn to be meek and humble of heart ! I unite all my actions and sufferings . . ." (as above).

AT TWO O'CLOCK (MORNING).

Jesus accused of blasphemy by Caiphas.

Adore Jesus as the teacher of truth, who prompted by love, suffered this great humiliation.

" O my Lord Jesus Christ, blessed be the hour in which Thou wast pleased to be delivered up to the fury of Thy malignant enemies ! Grant that through love of Thee I may sincerely humble myself. I unite all my actions and sufferings . . ." (as above).

AT THREE O'CLOCK (MORNING).

While Jesus suffered ill treatment in His prison, He has the sorrow to be thrice denied by Peter.

Contemplate and be amazed at the deep sorrow of Jesus Christ; ponder over His utter abandonment by His disciples, the cowardice of St. Peter, and the malice with which the Jews blindfold Our Lord's eyes, strike and deride Him.

" O my Lord Jesus Christ, blessed be the hour in which by a compassionate glance Thou didst touch the heart of Thy disciple ! Penetrate my heart also, I beseech Thee, with sentiments of love and of contrition for my sins. I unite all my actions and sufferings . . ." (as above).

AT FOUR O'CLOCK (MORNING).

Jesus led before the High Council and declared guilty of death.

Admire the humility and patience of our divine Saviour.

" O my Lord Jesus Christ, blessed be the hour in which Thou didst silently take upon Thyself the great ignominy of being looked upon as a blasphemer and a criminal guilty of death ! I adore Thee, O eternal Word, and unite all my actions and sufferings . . ." (as above).

AT FIVE O'CLOCK (MORNING).

Jesus is led before Pilate and accused anew.

Salute Our Lord, and adore Him as your Teacher, Saviour, and King.

" O my Lord Jesus Christ, blessed be the hour in which for the love of us Thou wouldst suffer this new ill treatment ! I unite all my actions and sufferings . . ." (as above).

AT SIX O'CLOCK (MORNING).

Jesus stands before Herod, who causes Him to be clothed with a white garment and to be treated as a fool.

Adore the Son of God, who on this occasion appears to be deprived of His divine attributes.

" O my Lord Jesus Christ, blessed be the hour in which Thou wouldst be satiated with contumely ! May it be a consolation to me when I shall meet with contempt for Thy sake ! I unite all my actions and sufferings . . ." (as above).

AT SEVEN O'CLOCK (MORNING).

Jesus led back to Pilate.

Adore the Heart of Jesus; although it is the inexhaustible treasury of every good, and open to all, men know it so little.

" O my Lord Jesus Christ, blessed be the hour in which Thou wouldst suffer this most injurious slight ! Disengage my heart from all earthly

things. I unite all my actions and sufferings . . ."
(as above).

AT EIGHT O'CLOCK (MORNING).

Jesus tied to the pillar and cruelly scourged. His blood flows on all sides.

Admire the unbounded love of our dear Saviour; each and every one of His wounds gives testimony of it.

" O my Lord Jesus Christ, blessed be the hour in which, being torn by the scourges, Thou didst shed Thy precious blood for the expiation of my sins ! I unite all my actions and sufferings . . ."
(as above).

AT NINE O'CLOCK (MORNING).

Jesus crowned with thorns and brutally ill-treated by the soldiers.

Adore the divine King of your heart suffering this cruel torment for you.

" O my Lord Jesus Christ, blessed be the hour in which for our love Thou wouldst suffer this painful crowning with thorns ! Wound my heart with sorrow and contrition for my sins. I unite all my actions and sufferings . . ." (as above).

AT TEN O'CLOCK (MORNING).

Jesus sentenced to death by Pilate and delivered up to the cruelty of the Jews.

The Holy of holies is treated like a malefactor,

and led to Calvary with His cross on His shoulders. Adore Him.

"O my Lord Jesus Christ, blessed be the hour in which for the love of us Thou wouldst be condemned to death and given into the hands of Thy cruel enemies. Thou then didst go along the way to Calvary laden with a heavy cross, in order to help me to bear mine with patience. I render Thee thanks for it and unite all my actions and sufferings . . ." (as above).

AT ELEVEN O'CLOCK (MORNING).

Jesus stripped of His clothes and fixed to the cross.

Adore the divine Lamb which is being sacrificed on the altar of the cross.

"O my Lord Jesus Christ, blessed be the hour in which Thou wast stripped of Thy clothes and slain as a lamb for the sins of the world ! Give me a heart capable of corresponding with so great a love. I unite all my actions and sufferings . . ." (as above).

AT NOON.

Jesus prays for His murderers, and promises paradise to the good thief.

Adore the divine Shepherd, who giveth His life for His sheep.

"O my Lord Jesus Christ, blessed be the hour in which Thou wouldst become an expiatory sacrifice for us ! Let Thy cross mitigate the rigor of

Thy judgment and comfort my soul in the hour of death. I unite all my actions and sufferings . . ." (as above).

AT ONE O'CLOCK (AFTERNOON).

Jesus commends His spirit into the hands of His Heavenly Father, confides His holy Mother to John, His beloved disciple, and the disciple to His holy Mother.

Admire the perfect abandonment of our most holy Redeemer on the cross. Thank Him unceasingly for the love which moved Him to confide us to His divine Mother in the person of St. John.

" O my Lord Jesus Christ, blessed be the hour in which Thou didst make known Thy will that Mary should become our Mother ! Grant that her love and Thine may inflame my heart to love you in return ! I unite all my actions and sufferings . . ." (as above).

AT TWO O'CLOCK (AFTERNOON).

Jesus cries aloud: " My God, my God, why hast Thou abandoned Me ? " And then He says: " I thirst ! " And after having tasted of the vinegar: " It is consummated ! "

Admire the unshaken patience of the Son of God, and compassionate His burning thirst for our salvation.

" O my Lord Jesus Christ, blessed be the hour in which Thou wouldst give us so touching an example of resignation in all kinds of suffering; of zeal for the salvation of souls, and of accomplishing the will of Thy heavenly Father ! I unite all my actions and sufferings . . ." (as above).

AT THREE O'CLOCK (AFTERNOON).

Jesus calls out with a loud voice, bows His head, and gives up the ghost.

Admire the last sigh of thy divine Saviour and the sacrifice which He makes of Himself for our salvation on the cross.

" O my Lord Jesus Christ, blessed be the hour in which Thou wouldst die for us in order to accomplish the great work of our redemption ! I unite all my actions and sufferings . . ." (as above).

AT FOUR O'CLOCK (AFTERNOON).

A soldier pierces the side of Jesus with a lance. Joseph and Nicodemus take the sacred body down from the cross and lay it in the arms of His afflicted Mother.

Adore this holy wound in the side from which blood and water flow.

" O my Lord Jesus Christ, blessed be the hour in which by this wound in Thy side Thou wouldst open to us Thy sacred heart, the source of salvation and of grace ! Let the unction of Thy grace flow down upon us through the hands of Mary, whom Thou hast given us as a Mother. I unite all my actions and sufferings . . ." (as above).

AT FIVE O'CLOCK (AFTERNOON).

Jesus wrapped in a linen cloth and laid in the sepulchre.

Adore Jesus Christ, who remains on our altars in a state similar to that in which He lay in the sepulchre.

" O my Lord Jesus Christ, blessed be the hour when, in order to be buried, Thou wouldst be given into the hands of Joseph and Nicodemus ! This reminds me of the generous love with which Thou givest Thyself into the hands of Thy priests in the holy Sacrifice of the Altar, in order to satisfy all our wants.

" O my Jesus, let me have a share in the compassion of Thy holy Mother; give me the courage, like these two disciples, to overcome all human respect; but especially give me the burning love of St. Mary Magdalen, that I may seek Thee until I have found Thee, who hast risen and diest now no more. I unite all my actions and sufferings ..." (as above).

Examples.

On his fortieth birthday *Frederick Ozanam,* founder of the Associations of St. Vincent of Paul, which are now spread over the whole world, wrote the following in his diary: " Thou hast, O my God, given forty years of existence to a creature who entered this world sickly and weak, and would ten times have been doomed to death but for the tenderness and intelligence of a father and a mother who ten times saved me. When at seven years of age a typhoid fever brought me to death's door, was it not to the intercession of St. Francis Regis that my mother ascribed my recovery? Hast Thou not cured me of the debility of my youth, which was a subject of uneasiness to my father? When at the outset of my career I was suddenly attacked by a serious disease of the throat, didst Thou not then cure me? Hast Thou not given me the joy to publish what I considered to be the truth? And last of all, five years ago didst Thou not recall me to life, granting me time to do penance for my sins and to amend?" During his long sufferings, the spirit of thanksgiving which had always animated him never left him for an instant.

His illness increasing, he went with his family to San Jacobo near Leghorn at the beginning of May, 1853. He was hardly able to read or write; but till the end of July he could not be prevented from going daily to hear Mass at the neighboring church, and in the evening to walk for a short time by the seashore. The people of the neighborhood showed the greatest attention to "the saintly stranger." They brought him flowers, for which he had always had a liking, also fruits and ice to cool the heat of the fever. At times he might be seen pacing the terrace before his house, as any longer walk had now become impossible. On the 15th of August, the Feast of the Assumption, his longing for the house of God was greater than his physical powers. "If it is to be my last

going out on earth," said he to his wife, " let it be
to the house of the Lord on this day; " and supported by her arm, he set out on his way to church.
The villagers stood outside the church, and all,
men, women, and children, gave him the most
cordial greeting. The sympathy of the people
moved him to tears. At the same time the aged
curé of Antignano was seriously ill. But as soon
as he heard that Ozanam was coming to church and
had asked to have holy communion before Mass,
the first word he said in reply was: " Help me to
get up: I must give it to him; no other shall have
this privilege." So he allowed himself to be
dressed, and then dragged himself painfully to the
church, where he gave holy communion to both
Ozanam and his wife. It was his last ecclesiasti-
cal function in life, as it was also Ozanam's last
visit to a church.

From this time the sick man spoke very little;
and when he did, it was only of sin and of the
punishment it deserves. A person one day re-
marking that he had not been so great a sinner,
he replied with as much seriousness as decision:
" Child, you do not know what the sanctity of
God is." The greater his bodily weakness became,
the more he prolonged his usual meditations.
When in greatest pain they had but to read to him
a few verses of Holy Scripture, especially from the
Book of Job, and he regained calmness and resignation. His mind, however, had lost nothing of its
buoyancy, and he now made use of it only to con-
centrate it on things eternal. Nothing was al-

lowed to interrupt his intimate intercourse with his God. " One evening," his brother Charles tells us, " finding him downcast, I tried to dispel the cloud. ' Alas, my dear brother,' said he, ' I am sad, there is no doubt; but it is a sadness bitter and sweet at the same time. When I think of my sins, and that they are the cause of the sufferings of Our Lord, I cannot refrain from tears;' and then he wept abundantly."

At the end of August, Ozanam longed to return to France, in order to die in his native country. When everything was ready for leaving, he wished to go and look out on the sea once more. Supported by his wife and one of his brothers he tottered to the terrace. Here he stood for a moment, with his gaze fixed on the billows which broke on the beach. Then he bared his head in the sunshine, lifted it up, and said aloud: " O my God, I thank Thee for the sufferings and tribulations Thou hast sent me in this place; receive them as an expiation of my sins ! " Then he turned to his wife, saying: " I would have you thank God with me for my sufferings; " and falling into her arms, he said: " I also bless Him for the consolations He has bestowed upon me." Then they took him on board the vessel, where a bed had been prepared for him. The voyage did him some good; and when the coasts of Provence came in sight, his joy was great to see his native country again. He summoned all his strength to get up when the boat entered the harbor of Marseilles.

However, the ultimate wish of his heart to return to Paris was not gratified. He suddenly became so weak that to continue the journey was out of the question. With full consciousness he received the sacraments of the Church, and he himself answered the prayers of the priest. But soon after he fell into a doze, and when he awoke he stretched out his hand either to thank or to bless. He heard with joy of the great interest which the members of the Association of St. Vincent at Marseilles took in him; and when his brother encouraged him to confide in God, he answered: " Why should I fear Him ? I love Him so much ! " On the evening of the Nativity of Our Lady, September 8th, his last hour arrived. He suddenly opened his eyes, lifted up his arms, and cried with a loud voice: " My God, my God, have mercy upon me ! " These were his last words.

A young *lady* of education and rank, who lived in affluent circumstances and was devoted to her husband and children, became consumptive. This disease at the end of *six months*, after causing her severe suffering, reduced her to the last extremity. Convinced of the certainty of her approaching end, she by constant efforts had attained a perfect resignation to the will of God, making freely to Him the sacrifice of herself and all that was dear to her on earth. Thus she knew no other fear than that of giving way to impatience—a fear which was well grounded on account of her irritability. Her vigilance over herself and her delicacy of conscience went so far as to take for signs of impatience even the smallest utterance of pain, such as the natural moan when tossing from one side to another. " Suffer *what* God wills, and as long as He wills, if only I am able to suffer *as* God wills." This was her watchword to the end. Therefore in her greatest sufferings she used to say: " God is *so* good "—emphasizing the word *so* with peculiar and touching fervor. On being asked how she was, she invariably answered: " Well; " or, " If I only preserve patience; " or, " If God only leaves me patience; " " God be praised for giving me patience." In her last days her patience rose to a perfect renouncement of her own will. She asked for nothing, took what was given to her, and all with cordial thanks. She was like a docile child.

The sight of her total abandonment to God, of her intimate union with Him by faith and love, filled every one with holy reverence. A short while before her end, she said with the most yearning desire: " Oh, if Jesus did but come ! If He would come soon ! " Yet she at once turned to her director, asking him with some uneasiness whether it was right for her to have such an intense desire; if this were not impatience. He quieted her, and said that such a desire was undoubtedly pleasing to Our Lord, whereupon she answered: " But I should wait until He comes." " Well, then—do both," he replied; " say with heartfelt desire: ' Lord Jesus, do come quickly ! ' and add with perfect resignation: ' As long as Thou wilt.' " " As long as Thou wilt," she repeated. Shortly after she expired gently and calmly, saying with a celestial smile, even in the arms of death, " He is very near me ! "

Princess Amalia of Gallitzin had for many years sought her happiness far from God in the enjoyment of the world, but her heart found in it nothing but vanity and vexation of spirit. Now God sent her a severe illness, and for three years she carried on a constant struggle within herself, till at length she threw herself into the arms of her Saviour and heavenly Physician. On the feast of St. Augustine she made a general confession, and thenceforward she sought her consolation and strength in religion only. For the space of twenty years she had to suffer much from bodily complaints, and to battle against a distressing melancholy. However, she looked for no human consolation, patiently bearing her cross after her divine Saviour. Her resignation to the divine will was especially a matter of great edification during the two months of her last illness. From the 2d of March, 1806, she had to keep her bed constantly, without being able to remain up even for a few minutes. Before this she had suffered acute pain only when she trod heavily, but now she could neither sit nor stand without suffering intensely. However violent these throes were, causing her at times to cry out, they were, as she said, more supportable than the increasing interior tension which was the consequence of dropsy and caused her great anxiety. Besides this she was seized by a painful vomiting, which set in about every three or four hours, and was most distressing for her attendants to behold. For several years she had, according to the advice of St. Francis of Sales, whom she had chosen for her special guide, addressed the following request to God: " Lord, I will not make any use of my own will; do Thou will for me, I beseech Thee, what is most pleasing to Thee !" In her last illness she at various times said to Overberg: " It seems to me impossible to will anything else but what God wills; for it is as clear to me as the sun that what He wills is best." She never expressed any desire to live longer nor even to die in order to be with Christ, although this was the single aim of all her wishes. At length, intimately united to Jesus by suffering, she died a gentle and holy death, April 27, 1806.

CHAPTER VI.

Assistance in Death.

THE most important epoch in human life is undoubtedly the hour of death, because upon it eternity depends. It sometimes happens that a sick man expressly asks his nurse to inform him if his death is near, because he has yet something on his mind which he wishes to reveal only later on. Do not, then, neglect in good time, yet cautiously, to acquaint the patient that his case is very dangerous, and that the doctor has no hope of his recovery. Many sick people even on their death-bed have made invalid confessions, not deeming themselves so dangerously ill, and therefore thinking they would make a good confession later, before their death. In such a case it is a sacred duty not to deceive the sick man, but earnestly to exhort him to regulate the affairs of his conscience. Sometimes it may even be advisable prudently and discreetly to give him to understand that if his mind be not yet entirely at peace the priest may be called in again, or even another priest.

When the sick man, after receiving the sacraments, is near his end, you must endeavor by every means in your power to secure his perseverance in good dispositions to the end. Exert yourself to make him turn away entirely from temporal cares and worldly things, in order to occupy himself solely with God and his salvation. That nothing may prevent him from doing this, endeavor to bring him to such a disposition of mind as to be ready for the love of God to leave everything, even those persons who are nearest and dearest to him, such as father, mother, wife, children, etc. Resignation, patience, confidence, charity, and the like good dispositions should be preserved and reanimated in the dying man; but especially he should be strengthened against the assaults of the devil, which at the approach of death are frequently far more violent than before.

Take good care that the sick man does not receive too many visits; these visits only worry him and rob him of the repose and recollection so necessary in order to enable him to occupy himself with God and to prepare himself for a happy end; visitors too often flatter the poor sufferer with false hopes of recovery, in consequence of which his good dispositions, especially his perfect resignation to the will of God, are weakened. Be mindful also that the sick man has a crucifix, a picture of Our Blessed Lady, of St. Joseph, or other saints near at hand, so that his eyes may constantly meet pious objects and that from time to time he may kiss or press them to his heart with love and confidence, which will greatly console and strengthen him.

If the sick man during life was invested with the scapular, be careful to let him wear it and continue to wear it until death; for it happens but too frequently that in the time of illness it is put aside through inattention, and that thus many graces and indulgences are lost. But if he has never been invested, inform the priest that, according to circumstances, he may give him the scapular.

If it has not already been done by the priest, explain to the sick man the meaning of the General Absolution, that he may gain the plenary indulgence attached to it; remind him also to direct his attention that he may gain the other indulgences connected with the Confraternities to which he belongs, as also those attached to the possession of blessed rosaries, crosses, and medals. In order to gain these indulgences granted for the hour of death, besides the reception of the sacraments and a willing acceptance of death, no special prayers are prescribed except the invocation of the most holy name of Jesus either orally or, if this is not possible, at least in the heart. (See page 186.)

Do not neglect frequently to sprinkle the bed and room of the sick man with holy water, this being an extraordinary defence against the assaults of the evil one.

Short but earnest and heartfelt prayers, ejaculations, and affections are the best encouragements for persons seriously ill, and especially for the dying. Say them slowly, in a gentle, devout tone, distinctly, emphatically, pronouncing the separate syllables, making frequent pauses, by way of rest for the sick man and to enable him to think over what is said. Moreover, remind the patient that it is not absolutely necessary to repeat the words orally; if this tires him, let him repeat them in his heart. Continue with these suggestions at least from time to time, even though he appear already to have lost consciousness, for this loss is often only apparent, the hearing being the last sense to refuse its services to the dying.

Do not allow many persons to be admitted into the room, as this would make the air bad and heavy and might give uneasiness to the dying person. It is far better for visitors to remain in the adjacent room and there pray in a low voice. The nearest relatives, above all, should be kept away when there is fear that by their too loud manifestations of grief they might disquiet the dying person or disturb the priest in his holy functions. Keep a window half open, or air the room a little from time to time. Now and then give some refreshment to the sick man, and, if he is unable to swallow, frequently moisten his lips and temples with wine, or with vinegar mixed with water.

Examples.

St. John Berchmans on the eve of his death asked the assisting priest not to leave him, because that night the decisive hour would come and there would be a hard battle with Satan.

At the words " Monstra te esse matrem " Berchmans suddenly stopped short, raised himself in his bed, and cried: " Pray, pray ! the attack of the infernal spirits is at hand and I am in dread of it." The priest encouraged him and he became quiet.

At midnight he suddenly and hastily lifted himself up from his couch; his look was directed towards heaven, and, while his lips were quivering and his countenance was filled with horror, he cried with a heart-rending voice: " No, no, this I will not do ! O Lord, I will not offend Thee ! O Mary, no, I will not offend thy Son ! God preserve me from such an evil ! Rather die ! Yes, rather die a thousand times, a hundred thousand times, a million times rather die ! " For a long time he continued crying: " A million times die, a million times die ! " His loud cries being heard by those in the adjacent room, they hastened to his help, fell on their knees, and began to pray. Suddenly the saint turned to the side of the bed, and cried with a firm and courageous voice: " Ah, Satan, begone ! " Then taking hold of his crucifix, his rosary, the little book containing the rules, and a reliquary, and showing them to his invisible enemy, he said: " Those are my weapons ! " And contemplating them one after the other, like a soldier viewing his armor, he said to himself: " What should I fear ? This cross—it has triumphed over hell ! The rosary—the Virgin Mother has crushed the serpent's head ! My rules —they are appointed to destroy the kingdom of Satan. These relics—the saints have triumphed over Satan ! "

After having received absolution once more, he remained thus resting on his knees till about five o'clock; only the motion of his lips showed that he had not lost consciousness, and that he joined in the prayers of the bystanders.   After some time he once more devoutly pronounced the names of Jesus and Mary, and his beautiful soul left its mortal frame, to be forever united with God and his blessed Mother.

Bernadette Soubirous, who had been favored with the apparition of Our Lady at Lourdes, afterwards entered the convent of the Sisters of Charity at Nevers, where she died April 16, 1879.   Besides an attack of asthma, she had much to suffer from a swelling of the knee and from caries.   The poor patient was obliged to remain in her bed or an armchair, being, like her divine Spouse, fixed as it were on the cross.   The violence of pain frequently wrung from her a cry which she was unable to repress, but which she at once changed into a fervent prayer, saying with energy: " My God, I offer it to Thee !   My God, I love Thee ! Yes, my God, I will have it so; I will have Thy cross ! "

Easter Tuesday was the day of her spiritual agony; the devil sorely tormented her, as he had assailed Jesus in the Garden of Olives and many of the saints.   During the night she was heard to exclaim several times: " Begone, Satan ! "   In the morning she told her confessor that the devil had caused her great terror, but that all had vanished upon her pronouncing the name of Jesus.   The combatant of Christ having strengthened herself with the holy Viaticum, the fight recommenced. In the evening she said to Sister Natalia, the second assistant, in whom she placed special confidence: " O my dear Sister, I am afraid—I am afraid ! " Being encouraged by her, she replied: " Alas ! I have received such great graces; but I fear I have benefited by them too little."

On Easter Wednesday, at one o'clock, she asked to see her confessor, wishing to cleanse her soul once more by the Sacrament of Penance. Pope Pius IX. by a special brief having granted her his blessing for the hour of death, she held the diploma in her hand while the blessing was given to her, and invoked the name of Jesus in order to gain the plenary indulgence. An instant later she said with ardor: " My God, I love Thee with all my heart, with all my soul, and with all my strength." Those present began the prayers for the dying, in which she joined with a faint yet audible voice.

The bystanders remarked with emotion that every now and then the dying Sister raised her large eyes and gazed intently at the crucifix which hung upon the wall. When it was placed in her feeble hands she took hold of it convulsively and pressed it closely to her heart, as if she would engrave upon it the print of the crucifix. A little before three o'clock, as Sister Natalia entered the room, Bernadette held out her arms to her and said with entreaty: " Oh, assist me, assist me ! pray for me ! " Then she asked pardon once more from the surrounding Sisters for having given them so much trouble. In her Saviour crucified she now sought all her strength; and taking up her crucifix with fervor she slowly kissed the five holy Wounds. Twice did Bernadette lisp the Hail Mary, which she had so often prayed at the grotto and which now the Sisters repeated to her. The third time she said: "Hail Mary, Mother of God—" She could go no farther, but, inclining her head, gave up her pure soul into the hands of God.

In order to be able to assist effectually the dying man in his last moments, when he is in particular need of spiritual help, it is of great importance to know the *signs of approaching death.* According to St. Alphonsus the most evident signs are: when the breath is gradually growing shorter; when in respiring the breast heaves more slowly and with greater difficulty; when the pulse is slower, stops at intervals, or fails altogether; when the eyes are deeply sunken and glassy, or remain wide open and stare in a vacant manner. Other signs of approaching death are: when the sick man begins to breathe through his nose; when the lips are growing white; when the hands begin to tremble and, as it were, grope about; when the finger-nails become blue; when the face appears quite changed and of a yellowish-blue color. Other prognostics are: when the body in the region of the heart is very warm, but the extremities, such as the hands and feet, are cold, and at times, also, when the face is covered with a cold sweat and the breath becomes cold and offensive.

Signs of immediate death are: slow pulsation with long intervals between the beats; setting of the teeth; sinking of the jaw-bone; saliva trickling out of the mouth, the eyes filling with a tear-like moisture; distortion of the eyes and mouth, and a peculiar low moan or sob which at times becomes audible.

In persons suffering from inflammation of the lungs the approach of death is indicated by their heavy breathing and by their lips turning blue. When dropsical persons are dying, the pulse ceases, while the gasping increases and the mouth is filled with phlegm. In those who suffer from consumption, asthma, and constriction of the larynx, from vomiting, rheumatism, and catalysis, or from wounds, it sometimes happens that very few of the above-mentioned symptoms appear.

During the death agony the dying person must not be moved, for fear of hastening death. Nor is it expedient to touch his hands and feet frequently, to see whether they are already cold, for this might easily disquiet him.

When the dying man is near his end, light the death candle. A wax candle specially blessed for this purpose is the best; but as such a candle is to be found in very few houses, it is well for the nurse to have one in readiness. A taper blessed on Candlemas-day is most appropriate, because it reminds us of the joy with which holy Simeon intoned his "Nunc dimittis," when he received the

Saviour, the Light of the world, into his arms. The prayers of the Church most fittingly implore protection against the prince of darkness, who exactly at the moment of death exerts all his power, knowing as he does that his time is short. Let this candle be placed near the sick man, or, in case he is very near death, put it into his hand as a sign that he wishes to depart this life in the light of the Catholic faith, and recite the suitable prayers (see Part III.). Arrange the candle in such a way that the light shall not fall straight into the dying man's eyes, which would be hurtful to him. When the agony draws to its end, the *Recommendation of the Departing Soul* (Commendatio animæ) as used by the Church is to be said kneeling; in the absence of a priest one of the bystanders may do this.

When the sick man appears to have expired, hold a mirror or a feather before his mouth and see whether the glass becomes clouded or the feather moves. If neither takes place, one can with tolerable certainty assume that death has supervened. The same assumption holds when the body is particularly heavy or shows gray or blue stains, as also when the heart is perfectly cold and a putrid odor is emitted, or when a peculiar moisture flows from the mouth or nose. If such signs are perceptible, kneel down and say the prayer: " Go forth," etc., and sprinkle the corpse with holy water. Exhort the assistants at once to join with you in saying the Litany for the Dead, or the like.

The clothes of the corpse should not be changed before it has grown cold; and even then it should be left lying in the bed, and as a rule should not be undressed and washed before the lapse of twenty-four hours. Lastly, in the opinion of experienced doctors it is a great mistake to tie up the mouth with a handkerchief, as is frequently done after death, because in case of a trance the returning respiration might thereby be prevented. If possible, the corpse should not be left alone for the first twenty-four hours, and the watching should continue until certain signs of death appear; such signs are, according to the declaration of physicians, the rigidity of death and dissolution.

A crucifix and a rosary are usually placed in the hands of deceased Catholics; besides this a burning candle, a crucifix, and a holy-water font with asperges are placed near the corpse.

SEVERAL PARTICULAR KINDS OF SICK-NURSING.

Care of the Sick in their Own Dwellings.

RELIGIOUS are obliged to go to all the sick to whom they are sent by their superiors, no matter whether they be rich or poor, Catholic or not, and whatever illness they may have, even though the nurses might fear contagion for themselves. What more beautiful death could they die than that of martyrs to charity ! Nevertheless we must not tempt God by neglecting simple precautions which are within our reach. We are by no means absolute masters and proprietors of our life and health; we have to make use of these gifts, entrusted to us by God, according to His will, and in such a manner as to be at all times ready to make the entire sacrifice of them in case He should require it.

If you are sent to a sick man, and if time permits, first of all make a visit to the Blessed Sacrament, invoke the protection of your divine Saviour, of the Blessed Virgin, of St. Joseph and your holy patrons, and then go on your way with confidence in God and strong in the power of holy obedience.

It is quite right to inform the parish priest of

the name of the person whom you have undertaken to nurse, and to ask his advice what line of conduct to follow. This is particularly advisable if you have non-Catholics to take care of, especially in the case of mixed marriages.

After a few days, a week at most, give a faithful account to your superiors of the circumstances in which you are placed, that they may decide whether due allowance is made for all the requirements of the case, or whether, perhaps, a change be desirable or necessary.

Be strictly attentive to whatever the doctor prescribes when visiting; but if several physicians are attending, retire as soon as they begin their consultation, unless they ask you to do otherwise.

In well-to-do families it will be enough for you to limit yourself to the service of the sick person, and to spend the rest of your time in manual work. But, if required, you may also go to the kitchen or elsewhere to get what is necessary and to prepare the requisite food. However, do not converse with the servants more than is necessary, and avoid every sort of familiarity with them; beware of listening to their complaints against their masters, and of secretly accepting food or drink from them.

As a rule do not undertake night-watching more than twice a week. Be relieved, if possible, at midnight, and be mindful on the following day to rest at least six hours. Make provision that another reliable person, man or woman, shall take care of the sick person in your absence.

When the illness proves to be dangerous, take all reasonable precautions that the sick man may receive the sacraments; if he objects to this, have recourse to prayer, consult your superiors, and inform the priest of the danger in which your patient is placed.

When for the alleviation of the sick man amusing conversation appears to be advantageous, let the infirmarians willingly join in it, but in such a manner that the discourse remains within the bounds of religious gravity. If the patient wishes, they can, with the physician's consent, read a devotional book to him. If other works are presented to them for reading aloud, they should, if they do not know them, ask the advice of the priest or of some other experienced and reliable person. This chiefly applies to tales which, although contained in Catholic periodicals, in many cases are not fit to be read by religious. How long the reading should last is for the doctor to determine. It is in no case allowable to read to non-Catholics from their prayer and devotional books or other religious writings. The same is to be said of such periodicals, publications, or journals whose tendency is decidedly hostile to the Church.

At all times avoid angry discourses and debates on matters of religion; if you are frequently importuned in this way, discreetly but decisively declare that under such circumstances you prefer to give up sick-nursing. Also it is never under any circumstances allowable to have anything to do with the religious functions of non-Catholic sextons or church-officers.

Try as far as possible faithfully to say the prayers and practise the holy exercises prescribed by the constitutions of your Order, and never to omit them through human respect, nor put off the reception of the sacraments beyond the fixed term. If your attendance upon a sick person is so continuously fatiguing as to prevent you from saying your office or other prayers and performing your holy exercises, do not neglect to make it known to your superiors and obtain a dispensation from them; in such cases endeavor to keep in the presence of God by frequent ejaculations, and to offer Him the hardships inseparable from nursing the sick.

If an invalid or his relatives give the religious something by way of a present, she cannot accept of it for herself and still less for her relatives, but only in the nature of and for her Community; and at her return she has at once to give it into the hands of her superiors, as well as the remuneration for the service of the sick.

At the request of the family, help to get the corpse ready for burial, but do not take part in any other of the arrangements for interment, but simply direct the relatives to apply to the parish priest.

When arrived at home, go to visit the Most Holy Sacrament and ask God's pardon for the faults you may have committed in your office. Then, if your superiors require, give them an exact account of the state of the sick man, of the service you have rendered him, and of the support he may perhaps still need.

Tending the Sick in Hospitals.

Before all things, it is absolutely necessary to keep strictly to the rules of the place, and neither to receive nor to dismiss any sick person without express leave on the part of the superiors. Moreover, beware, as much in your own interest as in that of religion and of your Order, of doing or permitting anything to be done contrary to the requirement of the civil authorities, or anything that cannot be publicly made known. In difficult and extraordinary cases consult your superiors and a prudent and experienced priest.

Let no one dare to perform operations or give medicinal prescriptions without the requisite authorization or sufficient knowledge; such matters must absolutely be left to the physician.

Try to obtain the confidence of the sick by an affectionate and delicate treatment, in order to gain them for God with greater facility; but at the same time carefully avoid too great familiarity. The greatest precaution and wisest reserve have to be adopted in relation chiefly to certain sick persons, because otherwise confidence may easily be abused and engender evil talk and even calumny.

If dissensions occur among the servants, they must be settled with the greatest calm in a separate place, without witnesses, and never in the presence of the sick.

Among the duties of nursing sick Catholics, the care of the spiritual welfare of the invalids should hold the first place. Therefore let the patients every day say a short morning and evening prayer, read from some good book, and if possible let it be done in common. And especially take care that the sick be provided in good time with the sacraments, chiefly on the eve of dangerous operations or at the beginning of such illnesses as are usually accompanied by delirium. When a sick man draws near his end, by no means leave him alone, but console and assist him with suitable exhortations and prayers.

As to the rest, in the case of the sick in hospitals observe as far as it is practicable what has been said in the previous chapter about sick-nursing in private houses.

Take care to prevent any loud noise in the wards in going to and fro, opening and closing the doors, and the like; if you speak to the other infirmarians, let it be in a low tone, so as not to be understood by the sick.

For the sake of order and punctuality it is highly advisable to have in each ward a slate on which may be written any necessary notes, together with the numbers of the respective beds.

When persons from outside come to visit the sick, be on your guard that they do not bring hurtful food or drink to the sick, as such imprudence might easily entail fatal consequences.

If practicable let there be a cupboard in one of the wards containing all the articles necessary for administering the sacraments. A key of the cupboard should be kept, if possible, not only by the chaplain, but also by others, such as the sacristan, the director, etc.; this precaution will prevent much annoyance.

The Care of the Sick on the Battlefield and in Ambulances.

The care of wounded and sick soldiers can be entrusted only to such persons as by their calm circumspection and resolute manner of acting, as also by their ability in dressing wounds, etc., are in a special manner qualified for this service. They must always carry with them some bandages and the most indispensable instruments.

On these occasions let religious most particularly endeavor by their outward demeanor to show themselves true to their calling and edify every one by their good example. Above all things they must be on their guard not to lose the spirit of mortification, and never let excessive exertion induce them to drink spirituous liquors immoderately. The hints previously given concerning their reserve in contact with the doctor, the inmates of the house, and the servants have still greater force here on account of the many and various persons with whom they have to deal. To religious placed in these unusual circumstances the greatest precaution and vigilance cannot be sufficiently recommended, since many a deplorable experience has but too well shown the necessity of it.

Although in the midst of these pressing and accumulated duties religious are legitimately dispensed from their usual prayers and exercises, yet, as soon as they find some leisure, they must not neglect by short ejaculations and pious reading to refresh and strengthen their soul.

Prudence requires that infirmarians in their letters, whether to their superiors or to other persons, should be very cautious, and especially refrain from complaints about insufficient support and similar matters. It is very easy for accounts of this sort when read by others to be wrongly interpreted, exaggerated, or even, without any bad intention, made known to the public.

The Care of Lunatics.

These unfortunate creatures having on account of their helpless state a peculiar claim to Christian charity, it is therefore an exceedingly meritorious work to devote one's self to their care through love of God, whose image they continue to be.

Three things there are which require the special attention of infirmarians: first, the *cure* of the invalids; secondly, *vigilance* over them; and thirdly, their *own personal safety*.

1. The *cure* of a diseased mind frequently de-

pends on the removal of bodily ailments. These ailments it is the office of the physician to cure; therefore his directions with respect to food, medicines, occupation, and recreation have most conscientiously to be executed. The taking of medicine must never be left to the invalid himself, but must be most strictly watched by the nurse, and if necessary given by her. If mental derangement is the consequence of a dissolute life, of evil habits, infidelity, despair, etc., it is necessary to give the priest an opportunity of speaking to the poor invalid in lucid moments and of arousing his conscience. The infirmarian should do this according to the direction given him by the priest; and above all he should take care to prevent the invalid from gratifying his passions and evil inclinations. Many insane persons have a very strong propensity to commit impure actions by themselves; and very experienced medical men declare that many of them would be cured of their insanity if they would overcome this vicious habit. For this purpose it is necessary to watch them very closely, especially if they were to commit such bad actions in presence of others whom they would perhaps induce to do the same.

Carefully avoid and remove everything that tends to foster their delusions and to rouse their passions. Also prevent their being exposed to the gaze of idle curiosity or mocked at by wanton levity. Listen to their irrational talk with visible indifference, and without ever attempting to convince them of their insanity by contradiction.

Let those who are at times sane, or who simply suffer from a fixed idea, be kept to the practice of their religious duties, especially to daily prayer.

To induce them to pray and to make a good general confession, provided it can still be done in lucid moments, are undoubtedly the greatest benefits that can be rendered to them. It often happens that at the hour of death reason returns to these unfortunate sufferers. Therefore avail yourself of this favorable time; let them make an act of contrition for their sins, recall to their memory the chief truths of faith, and if possible provide them with the sacraments.

2. The greatest *vigilance* by day and by night is to be maintained so that the invalids do not damage or spoil the clothing, beds, victuals, or other things, or injure themselves or others. Dangerous tools and instruments should only rarely be entrusted to them, and then under due superintendence.

These unfortunate persons are often inclined to commit suicide; the windows have therefore to be made fast, and if necessary provided with crossbars. For the same reason, cord, twine, string, materials for striking fire, and such like things should not be within their reach; in short, all possible precaution and watchfulness are in this respect necessary, as maniacs often display very extraordinary cunning to gain their ends.

Great prudence and skill are to be employed in the treatment of those who for a long space of time obstinately refuse to eat, and more especially of those who manifest the intention of starving themselves to death.

With regard to mad and raving persons, to whom food and drink are given in their rooms, minute attention must be paid whether they take food, and how much they consume.

This most indispensable superintendence must be carried on in such a manner as to be but little noticed by the patient himself, in order not to make him suspicious or induce him to have recourse to artifice. Every lunatic is to be treated with the esteem and attention due to his condition and circumstances in life, just as if he were not ill at all and as if apparently he were nursed more for recreation than for superintendence. The appellations "fool," "madman," "maniac," "madcap," etc., should never be made use of in his presence.

Heartfelt interest, gentle and affectionate treatment, together with a grave deportment are the essential requirements for a successful care of these unfortunate persons.

As soon as one of the patients is missed, it must at once be brought to the knowledge of the authorities of the house, that they may act accordingly.

3. *Not to expose yourself to unnecessary danger* while tending persons weak in mind, and especially madmen, caution is no less to be recommended than gravity and decision, although compassion and kindness must never be omitted. Never excite the patient's temper by invectives or

ill-timed jokes. If he talks nonsense or grows warm on one or another occasion, prudence requires that we should pacify him with kind and gentle words, and not excite him to anger by contradiction. If kind words are of no avail, it is a duty to keep strict silence and to recommend the matter to God.

Should refractory or frantic patients require to be treated with main force, it is by no means permissible to threaten them with it a long while beforehand. The application of strong measures must be made with the utmost forbearance, without abusing or offending the sick man either by word or deed.

While tending these unfortunate beings never manifest impatience, anger, embarrassment, fear, or the like; never lose your composure: on the contrary, as occasions call for it, display great intrepidity, presence of mind, and self-possession. To this end frequently consider that these outbursts of violence and frantic fits, these affronts and spiteful tricks, even the personal attacks on the sick-nurse, must be looked upon as the actions of men who are involuntarily urged to them by their malady, and who have lost their ordinary mental faculties.

Self-defence against the artful and violent attacks on the part of lunatics is of course not forbidden, but must only be employed in the most gentle and forbearing manner, to render the patient harmless.

APPENDIX.

A FEW OTHER EDIFYING EXAMPLES FOR THE SICK AND DYING.

Sick Children.

A LITTLE boy of seven years of age, the son of a smith named *Thiesing*, at Diepholz in Westphalia, in the winter of 1787 had one of his legs broken and crushed by a wooden sledge which passed over it. The child was carried home, and when the sad news was told to his sick mother she sprang out of bed and fainted away. During the painful operation which then took place the little boy kept perfectly quiet, folded his hands over his head, and did not give even the least utterance of pain. Those around him were astonished at so much firmness, and asked him if he did not feel most violent pains. "Oh, yes," he answered gently, "but I suppress them, that mother may not become worse." On the third day his physical sufferings appeared to overcome his fortitude; yet he manifested them only by a moan which was scarcely audible. Thus the poor child continued for a considerable time to suffer with incredible fortitude until he was cured. Later on the doctor told the mother how bravely the little one had borne his sufferings for her love; and this proof of tender filial affection so much consoled the mother's heart that her own recovery took place much sooner than was expected.

Frances O'Connor (d. 1835) at the age of twelve was sent to the convent of the Dames du Sacré Cœur at Paris to be educated. By prayer, mortification, and frequent acts of contrition she assiduously prepared for her First Communion, also by a serious combat against her evil inclinations, which were sensitiveness, laziness, and impatience. Meanwhile she was troubled by an obstinate and most painful sore on one of her fingers, and was afflicted with a weakness of the stomach which at times rendered her incapable of taking food. This gave rise to an irritability of the nerves which made it exceedingly difficult for her to keep her resolutions. With touching simplicity she then used to say to her mistress: " Ah, how I have to suffer, and how sorely I am tempted to give way to impatience ! " Being gently encouraged to bear her sufferings and to offer them to God, she said: " Ah ! indeed I will do so, in order to obtain the grace of a worthy First Communion, and above all the grace of contrition." And she kept her word. From excess of pain she was seen frequently to turn pale and to shed tears, but her sighs and moans were always intermingled with pious ejaculations, such as: " My God, I offer it to Thee ! " " My God, it is for Thee ! " During the six days' retreat in preparation for her First Communion, Frances was tormented by toothache and gout; she nevertheless persevered in all her spiritual exercises, and even tried to add voluntary mortifications. A cup of sugared milk being presented to her, she said: " Milk alone will do; what is the sugar for ? Ought I not to offer some little privations to our dear Lord, as I cannot pray on account of my pains ? " On the 31st of May, the eve of her First Communion, the fever which had set in the preceding nights considerably increased, and Frances had to go to bed without knowing whether on the following day she would be able to join her happy companions. Her anxiety, therefore, was exceedingly great, but she hoped all through the intercession of Mary. Indeed in the morning she felt a great deal better, and the physician declared she could get up and go to the chapel. At this good news heavenly joy lit up her face and made her strong enough to dress and to join her fellow pupils. Yet the solemnity was hardly at an end when the fever returned, obliging the poor child to return to bed. The illness made rapid progress and reduced Frances to a state of great weakness, while at the same time she could hardly take even the least refreshment. To change her linen or position almost invariably caused her fresh and great pain. But no sound of complaint came from her lips; she quietly smiled, and from time to time whispered some prayers. Her relatives coming to visit her and crying with compassion, she took hold of their hands and said tenderly: " Why are you sorrowful ? I am going to heaven, where I

shall pray for you." She never asked to have
her position changed, and when the Sister who
watched near her suggested this small alleviation,
she replied: " Jesus Christ was closely nailed to
the cross, so I also can remain as I am." After
several months of illness borne with quiet resignation Frances breathed her last, October 26, 1835.

poor Sick.

Pope Gregory the Great relates the following of a poor sick man named *Servulus,* who
from his very infancy, being troubled with gout,
could use neither his hands nor his feet. Pressed
by want, he allowed some good people to carry
him to the gate of the church of St. Andrew at
Rome, where he gratefully received the alms that
were given to him. If they were refused, or if
he met with rudeness and contumely, he did not
show the least impatience; and when evening
came, he was taken back to his poor mother and
brothers, to whom he gave the alms of the faithful, enjoining them not to keep more for themselves than they needed, and to distribute the rest
to the poor. However great his misery might be,
he daily returned thanks to God for his sufferings;
and when his end was drawing near, his pains
increased, but also his fervor in devoutly preparing for his last journey. Informing some poor
and pious friends of this good news, he entreated
them to sing psalms, and while they were singing
the praises of God he joyfully expired.

In the seventeenth century in the north of France lived a poor maid-servant, commonly called "the good *Armella*," who suffered from a variety of illnesses. At one time a continual fever combined with violent headache had so much exhausted her strength that she could no longer keep erect. However, her hard mistress took no notice of it, and, deeming her disease to be simply laziness, ordered her to carry manure into the garden. Armella shuddered at this command, but obeyed without reply, and, meek as a lamb, continued at her task for two days, suffering all the while from a frightful headache. It was to her as if the sharpest thorns were piercing her head; but as often as she carried a new load she would think of the crown of thorns of Jesus; and this reflection, as she herself confessed, rendered all her torments sweet and pleasant. She continually suffered from a very sharp pain all along the spine, which did not allow her to lie or to bend without suffering acutely. And yet this was the pain dearest to her, "because," said she, "my God and my Love, when carrying His cross, endured the most cruel pains in this very same place." Besides this she was frequently visited by violent colics. When the pain was at its height she invariably repeated the words: "Live Jesus and His pains!" In her old age one of her legs was fractured by the kick of a horse, while her other leg was attacked with running sores. Fifteen long months she was confined to her bed or to an armchair; only on Sundays and holidays she was carried to church; the rest of her time she spent in a corner of the kitchen and superintended the household, which had been entirely entrusted to her. Many people came to visit her to edify themselves by her rare patience and affable conversation. She begged them all to thank Our Saviour for the grace He had bestowed upon her by this illness. A priest one day telling her that he did not suppose she would die very soon, she readily and amiably replied: " God be praised, father; then I have some time more to suffer ! "

Courage in Bearing Illness.

At the age of seventy-four *St. Laurence Justinian,* being attacked by a violent fever and seeing his servants busy in preparing a bed for him, sorrowfully addressed them, saying: " What do you mean to do ? You only lose your time. My Saviour did not die on a bed, but on a cross." He insisted also on his being laid on straw. The heat of the fever tormenting him greatly, a refreshing drink was offered to him; but he declined it. " Let it alone; why should I refresh myself with a drink, while my Lord and Saviour in His mortal agony on the cross suffered thirst ? And besides, if we cannot bear this earthly thirst, how shall we be able to bear the flames of purgatory ? " Having to undergo a painful operation in his throat, his attendants and the doctor himself trembled before undertaking it. But the saint encouraged the operator, saying: " God knows how to help and to preserve. Only cut bravely ! " And then he prayed with all his heart: " O my Jesus, do let me have some share in Thy bitter passion ! " His illness increasing, the most heartfelt sympathy was shown him by his friends; but he exulted, saying: " Indeed, as I am too enfeebled to chastise my body, God's mercy takes my place and chastises me for my sins. Let Him be praised and extolled for it ! "

The last twenty years of the life of *St. Alphonsus of Liguori* were, so to say, a continual martyrdom, on account of the various painful maladies, such as fever, asthma, headache, etc., which he had to endure. In spite of his bodily sufferings, St. Alphonsus continued to visit his diocese, nay, even to write books, although he at times was troubled by such violent headaches that he had to cool his forehead with a piece of marble. A most obstinate rheumatism pervaded all the limbs of his body and at last settled on the cervical vertebra, which caused his head to be bowed down on his breast. Then the beard on the chin, continually pressing on his breast, gradually formed there a large wound, of which the saint never complained and which was perceived only by the pus discharging from it. During these illnesses he was at various times advised to call in several eminent doctors from Naples, but he would not consent to it. " My life is but of little importance," said he; " the physicians of Naples cannot work miracles either. I find myself quite well in the hands of God and of the doctors of this place."

Among other things he writes in his letters: "I continue to be in my neck-yoke without being able to stir, and I suffer in every part of my body. I suffer from neuralgia which will end only with my life; I cannot take a step or make a motion without pain; I keep my bed, but I thank God for giving me this favor."

Invalids Suffering with Joy.

The last year of his life, *Alphonsus Rodriguez,* a holy lay Brother of the Society of Jesus, was constantly confined to his bed, and the last three months he was obliged to lie continually on one side, without changing his position, which caused him a real martyrdom. Meanwhile he never ceased praying and invoking God, not for his recovery, nor for consolation, but for an increase of pains and for new sufferings. He only spoke of sufferings, and always with the same enthusiasm. "No one is happier," he exclaimed, "than he to whom God gives the grace patiently to suffer great pains. What better thing is there here below ? Did not the Eternal Father actually grant *this* to His Son ? Oh, if the angels and saints were capable of envy, they would be jealous of those who have much to suffer." This idea inspired him with the most sublime dispositions, and whatever he said in this regard was the result of his own experience, his patience being comparable to that of holy Job. When any one inquired about his health, he simply said: " With the grace of

God, it will go very well." On such occasions he liked best to repeat the little prayer which Our Lord Himself had taught him: "O Jesus and Mary, my sweetest love, grant me the grace that through love of you I may suffer, die, entirely forget myself, and wholly belong to you!" While his pains were increasing, he unceasingly went on praying: "Still more, O Lord, still more!" He frequently repeated the most sweet name of Jesus; and when the crucifix was presented to him tō kiss, he opened his eyes, ardently fixed them on the crucifix, and pronouncing with great fervor the most holy name of Jesus, surrendered his soul into the hands of God.

Maria of Escobar, a saintly virgin, was ill for thirty long years and all the time tormented with a variety of troubles and pains. Neither the physician nor any one else found means to help her. Moreover she had to battle with interior sufferings, being especially tempted against patience and resignation to the divine will. Yet Maria was almost constantly found to be cheerful, thanking God for these afflictions, and saying that these interior and exterior trials were dearer to her than all possible consolations. "Yes," said she, "if by moving one single finger I could free myself from all these afflictions and pains, I yet would not do so, because for these short and transitory sufferings I expect to find an everlasting reward in heaven."

Desire of Death.

We owe to a Catholic periodical the following
account by a parish priest: " A short time ago I
had the consolation of witnessing the death of a
simple, *God-fearing woman,* fifty years of age, who
from her childhood had had a singular devotion
to our blessed Lady. At the age of twenty, when
assisting at a mission, she made a vow of virginity
and most conscientiously kept her promise. After
having received the last sacraments she lived three
weeks, during which she several times received
holy communion. ' Father,' said she on one of
these occasions, ' there is still one doubt remaining to me. Is it right not to be afraid of death ? '
' This is quite right,' I replied. ' But I have so
great a desire to die ! ' ' You of course suffer great
pains,' I suggested, ' and you certainly may pray
to be released from them.' ' Alas ! no; but I
long so much to see Jesus ! ' and saying so, she
looked at a picture of Our Saviour hanging near
her bed. She repeatedly asked those around her
how much longer she had to live; and when, a few
hours before her end, she was told her divine
Saviour would soon call her hence, her languid
eyes lit up anew; a more joyful news could not
have been brought to her. ' I shall see Jesus !
I shall see Jesus ! ' she said again and again, while
heartfelt joy was reflected on her countenance.
And this expression of joy remained even during
her agony; and as if the parting soul had wished
to share with the body the happiness of beholding

Jesus, the expression of her countenance after her death was so sweet, lovely, and full of joy that all wondered and said they had never in life seen N. N. so beautiful and happy."

Another parish priest writes in *Notburga,* the above-mentioned periodical: "In passing by a farm, I was requested by its owner to visit his *maid-servant* Teresa, who was grievously ill. She had already received the last sacraments and was quietly awaiting her end. I sat down at her bedside and spoke to her words of consolation; I said among other things that a pious Christian ought not to fear death. She replied: 'Father, I am not afraid to die; I rejoice at the thought.' And when I asked the reason, she gave this beautiful answer, which remains indelible in my mind: 'I greatly rejoice to die, because I shall then see our dear Lord.' On the following day, Easter Monday, she breathed her last. This poor servant indeed had no cause to fear death, for she was a truly pious Christian. Teresa had served fourteen years in the same family; had diligently worked from morn to night; had talked little and lived in peace with her fellow servants. She had never suffered any one in her presence to speak improper language, and gave universal edification by her humble and modest behavior. Every Sunday and holy day she went a considerable distance to church to assist at Mass and hear a sermon, and every four or six weeks she devoutly received the sacraments. Before her death she bequeathed all her little possessions to the poor and to her fellow servants. The good farmer whom this worthy maid-servant had so long and so faithfully served has by no means forgotten her, and intends to have a Mass said each year on the anniversary of her death."

Grievous Temptations During the Agony of Death.

In the year 1859 *Father Hildebrand*, a pious Benedictine, died at Rome, aged twenty-eight years. Shortly before his death he turned to the left of his bed and said with great earnestness: "Audacious wretch that you are!" Those who were in attendance upon him, being in dread of the tempter, strengthened the invalid with blessings and prayers; they invoked Our Lady, St. Benedict, and especially St. Michael the Archangel, to whom he was greatly devoted. "St. Michael," he cried, "pray for me, combat for me! Thou wert at all times my protector, my guide; come with thy powerful aid!" Then he joyfully exclaimed, looking towards the side from which the temptation came: "St. Michael has overcome the infernal tempter!" However, another temptation, of distrust and despair, it appears, was in store for him. "What screams!" said he, again turning to the left, and then: "With your accursed 'If'!" Here he repeatedly crossed himself and then the bed. "They want to accuse me. I know I committed such faults every day, but I confide in Thee, O merciful Jesus!" Then he joined in saying the wonderfully efficacious prayer engraved on the medal of St. Benedict: " Vade retro, satana—Nunquam suade mihi vana—Sunt mala, quæ libas—Ipse venena bibas "; and then with uplifted hands broke out into fervent acts of contrition for the failings he had committed.

Concerning the agony of *Dr. Andrew Pankau,* professor of theology at Culm (d. 1871), we read in his obituary: " He summoned up all his remaining strength against the enemy of mankind, who in his last hours assailed him fiercely. In most dreadful anguish he raised himself up, held the coverlet with his arms—his hands already being dead—and called out many times with a more and more emphatic tone: "Tu ! Tu ! Tu !" Then he turned to the crucifix, exclaiming: " Thou Cross of truth ! " repeated nigh thirty times the names of Jesus, Mary, Joseph, always with a more earnest voice. All the bystanders were seized with terror at this hard struggle, which lasted about three minutes. At the words of the assistant priest: " St. Joseph, patron of our holy Church, pray for him " (which the dying man repeated with full consciousness together with the other prayers), the most perfect calm succeeded. By the names of Jesus, Mary, and Joseph the victory had been gained, the hard struggle was over, and, after half an hour's gentle breathing, the soul, disengaged from the body, went to receive the crown of victory.

ͪol̨ Deaths.

CHILDREN.

The well-known Abbé de Ségur writes: "I knew at Paris a good and innocent child of the name of Paul. From his fourteenth year he received holy communion every Sunday and at least once in the week besides. His life of perfect innocence was soon to be crowned by a holy death. After three or four months a rapid consumption brought him to the grave. On the eve of his death, May 8, 1862, I went to see him. There he lay on his bed almost breathless and lifeless, but in possession of perfect consciousness. 'Father,' said he, with an almost inaudible voice, 'I have something which troubles me.' 'What is it, my poor child? Is it a sin?' 'Oh, no, not that; but it seems to me as if I did not love Our Saviour enough.' I quieted him and gave him my blessing. The following morning his agony began, and his pious mother, kneeling at his side, expected him every minute to breathe his last. Then he suddenly looked up to heaven, extended his arms, while his countenance bore a seraphic expression impossible to describe; thus he remained a few moments with eyes and hands uplifted. 'What is the matter, child?' asked the wondering mother; 'what is it?' 'O dear mother!' said Paul in a clear and distinct voice, 'O dear mother! The beautiful Lady who comes towards me!' His arms sank down, his eyes closed; he was dead. His mother remained so convinced that the Blessed Virgin herself had come to take home the soul of her beloved son that she forgot all her sorrow, listening only to her faith; she sank down on her knees and prayed with a loud voice the Magnificat, ' My soul doth magnify the Lord.' She was worthy of her son."

The son of a good artisan of the district of Münster, who was only seven years of age, had caught a severe cold and for several days he had suffered from a bad cough, when one morning his father said to him: " Dear Henry, do not go out in this wind; you have a heavy cold; stay near the warm stove and write on your slate." The child readily obeyed, and began to write on his slate the little prayer well known by many children: " Dear God, I implore Thee to make me a virtuous child. But should I turn out otherwise, do take me home to paradise ! " Thus far Henry had written, when he complained of a very sore throat, asking his mother to let him go to bed. The fact was that the cold had brought on quinsy, which caused the little one to die on the evening of that very same day. His last sentence on the slate had been as it were a petition to the divine Friend of little children, who surely took His little favorite to paradise. This slate, with the petition of their beloved child so speedily granted, was kept by the afflicted parents as a precious souvenir of dear little Henry.

LAYMEN OF HIGH POSITION.

Charles Frederick of Savigny (d. 1875), president of the Centre Party, bore with truly Christian patience and resignation the severe sufferings which confined him to a sick-bed for the space of seven months. However deeply he might feel, he bore the trial with composure and resignation to the will of God. "God will provide," he said shortly before his death, with reference to this sacrifice. "He knows better what to do than I." The amiability and gentleness of his character did not abandon him even in the midst of exquisite pain. It would be difficult to find a man so charitable in his judgment regarding his opponents, so ready to pardon injuries however deeply he might feel them. On the very day of his death this noble trait of his character was thus expressed by his dying lips: "We must not bear ill-will to any one whatsoever." On Ash Wednesday he entered into the spirit of holy Church by the remembrance of death. After having received Extreme Unction, he kissed the priest's hand and said to the bystanders: "How beautiful this holy sacrament is!" Then he blessed his children, and his wife who had bestowed such loving care on him during his illness and who now knelt at his bedside, joining in his prayers. After having blessed his youngest child: "Now it is enough," said he, "now all is well!" These were the last words he uttered. Then gently and without agony he fell asleep in the Lord.

Herman of Mallinckrodt (d. 1874) was one of
the most valiant leaders of the Centre Party during the " Kulturkampf " in Germany. God called
him away from the field of action in the full vigor
of his life, at the age of fifty-three. At the close
of the Diet, while preparing for his return home,
he was seized by an indisposition which proved
to be an inflammation of the lungs. He at once
asked for and received the last sacraments and
said: " Like a child I longed so much to go home;
but if God decrees otherwise, I am satisfied. I do
not know what will happen, but, all things taken
into consideration, I can very well understand
why God calls me just at this time." He manifested the same absolute tranquillity as to the
event of his death. In the evening, a little after
having received the holy Viaticum, his wife
arrived, and brought him the greetings of his
children; he immediately inquired about their
health and various other matters. She at once
began herself to nurse her dearly beloved husband,
and never left his bedside. During the night, the
fever rapidly increasing, the sick man asked for
the indulgenced cross on his rosary. He kissed it
repeatedly and kept it in his hand. All the night
through he suffered great pain, but no complaint
came from his lips.

Towards midnight his state grew considerably
worse; the death-rattle became more audible; and
thus he lingered on till two in the afternoon, being
apparently unconscious. As his end seemed to be
approaching, a blessed candle was lighted, when

consciousness suddenly returned. Towards evening, when he was told that his sister Pauline of Mallinckrodt, the Superioress-General of the Sisters of Charity (Sœurs de la Charité chrétienne), was coming, he greatly rejoiced at the news. She arrived at half-past nine; and after having welcomed her most heartily, he said to her: " You might say the Rosary for me." The rest of the time he appeared frequently to be praying by himself, showing himself best pleased when the well-known indulgenced prayer, " Jesus, Mary, Joseph, to you I give my heart and my soul," was said to him. The delirium which at intervals had set in during the afternoon grew more intense at night. It was, however, interrupted by occasional moments of consciousness, and then he always appeared glad to see his family around him; he gave evidence of this by his look and the pressure of his hand. Thus he continued from Sunday till Tuesday morning. The clock having struck a quarter past ten, the sick man raised himself up in his bed, asked for his spectacles and writing materials, and then in a legible hand wrote the following words: " Truth ! liberty !" Then he paused an instant, lay down on his right side, and with his looks turned heavenwards, after a few heavy breathings, expired without agony.

PERSONS OF ROYAL BIRTH.

On the 19th of August, 1874, Her Royal Highness *Maria Immaculata de Bourbon* arrived at Pau. Hardly nine months had elapsed since her marriage with the nephew of Count de Chambord, when she was attacked with a serious disease of the lungs.

Perfectly conscious of the sad reality, she, on the very evening of her arrival, had an altar erected in her apartment, so as to enable her to hear Mass and receive holy communion on the following day.

The princess had always been looked upon as an angel of virtue by her family. The decision of her character, the solidity of her virtue, and her truly angelic innocence especially excited admiration. A few days before the feast of the Assumption she had asked for the grace to die on that day. However, the long-wished-for hour not appearing, she said mournfully: " O Mary, what a delightful day for death ! How happy I should deem myself to die on this festival ! " On the 20th of August, the princess, having received holy communion during the Mass, asked the priest, who was about to retire, to come again in the afternoon at three o'clock to hear her general confession. On his return he was introduced to Mlle. Lasserre, who said: " Father, the confession will not be long. The poor princess we have always looked upon as an angel." And so it proved; the confession was soon at an end, and the noble lady spent the rest of the day and the long, weary hours of the night in prayer, or in listening to pious reading in preparation for death, or in silently joining in the prayers made for her. All being ended, she felt very ill. " O father," she exclaimed, " how much I suffer ! I should not have thought it would last so long; pray to God to let me die." The priest reminded her that on the day following the Church celebrated the beautiful feast of the Immaculate Heart of Mary, and invited her to ask for the twofold grace, first, to be able once more to communicate and, secondly, to die on the feast of the Immaculate Heart of Mary. The sufferings of the poor victim grew ever more intense; nevertheless she continued calm and in prayer. As often as they ceased to pray she asked them to begin again.

As the pictures of St. Joseph and St. Aloysius were hanging over her bed, she at various times begged them to be handed to her to kiss. For more than two hours the princes and princesses recited in common several litanies; the sick lady made the utmost efforts to join in every word. Towards midnight the weakness visibly increased. She, together with all the members of the family, then received the body of Our Lord once more, and at the end of the thanksgiving she bade them all the last farewell. Not one tear moistened her cheek during this heartrending scene, nor did she betray the least emotion; everything breathed the peace and joyfulness of a soul wending its way to heaven.

Thus the first grace had been granted to her beloved child by our blessed Lady, and so also was the second. In the early morning of this beautiful day the agony began. Her voice was no longer heard, but one could see by the motion of her lips that she joined in the prayers of the dying which the royal family were reciting. From time to time the priest let her kiss the crucifix which she held in her right hand; each time her lips trembled with emotion, and she most devoutly kissed the five wounds. She wished frequently to be sprinkled with holy water, and made a sign when it had not been done for some time. The last moment approached. The priest once more recited in a loud voice an act of contrition, and gave the dying lady a last absolution. Then she turned towards a small statue of Our Lady of the Sacred Heart: it was the last glance. Then, with dim eyes, she once more kissed the crucifix with effusion. Her sufferings were at an end; her soul stood in the sight of God.

On the 7th of June, 1876, died one of the most worthy women of our day, *Queen Josephine of Sweden,* granddaughter of the first King of Bavaria, Maximilian I. On the night before the feast of the Ascension, May 24, 1876, this lady was attacked by a violent fever which the physician in ordinary, who was immediately called in, recognized to be a very dangerous incipient pleurisy and inflammation of the lungs. During her illness Josephine's subject of conversation was of God and of the love of our holy Redeemer, whose likeness, an Ecce Homo, was hanging at the top of her bed. After having received the last sacraments she pointed to her suffering Lord. " Here is the portrait of my dear Saviour whose blood was shed for the redemption of us all," she said, " but I—I have Himself to-day in the midst of my heart. What a beautiful day God has given me to see ! How little the great God makes Himself for our sakes, to make us little ones great ! " The Sister of Charity who had the happiness of nursing the good queen declared she had never seen any one dying so entirely free from temptation and uneasiness, and possessing such an unshaken confidence in God, as Josephine. No trace of agony or fear of death was to be detected on her beautiful countenance; gentle as a child in her mother's arms she lay within the arms of her loving God. On the night of her death, towards one o'clock, she was repeatedly heard to say in a singing tone: " Now I go home, I go home ! " Five minutes before her end, she exclaimed with a blissful, ecstatic smile on her dying lips: " I am happy, I am very happy ! " Then a few low, deep sighs, and the angels bore her soul before the throne of God.

PRIESTS.

Towards the end of September, 1883, *Professor Alban Stolz* felt so weak that he could no longer leave the house, and from the 2d of October he had constantly to keep his bed. Although he suffered no particular pains, yet the difficulty of breathing

increased. Meanwhile he repeatedly received
holy communion, and, being well aware that his
last hour was at hand, he asked for the last sacraments, which he received on the 12th of October
with perfect consciousness and singular devotion.
He commissioned his confessor to ask pardon of
all those whom he might ever have offended. On
Sunday, October 14th, he once more received holy
communion. From that time to his last moment
he was almost exclusively occupied with God in
prayer. After an apparent slumber, being asked
if he had slept well, he answered: " No, I conversed with God as well as I could."

At intervals he was seized with great fear with
regard to his salvation. The Sister of Charity
who had been serving him for many years, trying
to quiet him, he answered: " Sister, this is a thing
you do not understand; a priest has many things
to answer for." At another time, some one in-
tending to console him by alluding to the great
benefits he had spread through his words and writings, he replied: " I might have done still more
and worked better. And if we had done all, must
we not say with the apostles: ' Useless servants
are we' ? " (Luke xvii. 10.) Persevering in humility to the end, he placed his whole confidence
in the blood of Christ; he hardly ever let the crucifix go out of his hands, and innumerable times
kissed the wounds of his Saviour. As long as his
strength permitted he also frequently made the
sign of the cross. When the persons assembled
round his death-bed requested him to intercede

for them at the throne of God, he answered: " Yes, for all, all." Then he expressed his thanks for the services he had received, saying: " May God reward it all ! " These were his last words.

On November 22, 1866, a few hours before his death, the Reverend Dean of the Cathedral and Vicar-General *Lennig* at Mayence addressed the following words to a few friends assembled round his death-bed: " I am to appear before the tribunal of God, but I fear not. I am a poor sinner, and guilty of many, many faults; God never ceased to heap graces upon me. All my life long I have received great benefits. All sorts of good things have been given to me. I ought to have been far more thankful to God. I have not returned Him sufficient thanks. Now I surrender myself entirely to His divine will. I fear not. I confide in Jesus Christ, in the merits He has purchased for us on the cross, in His precious wounds and blood. I confide in the Most Holy Sacrament I received yesterday. I rely on the holy Mother of God; to her heart I always used to recommend myself. She will not forget me in death; she will intercede for me, and God will be gracious to me. I die in the faith of the holy Catholic Church. I have always been a faithful adherent to her; to her I must cling. Not one step to the right or left must one stray. I never wandered away from her. Therefore I do not fear. I confide in our dear Saviour, in His precious blood, in our holy Church and the sacraments, in the holy Mother of God and her intercession. Through her God will be propitious to me."

BISHOPS.

The sick-room of the late Archbishop of Cologne, *Clement Augustus* (d. 1845), was indeed a school where all might learn how to suffer and to die for God. At least once a day he would have the following beautiful verses read to him:

> " Like a sun-dial heavenwards set thy heart ;
> For, when the heart is set on God,
> It goeth with each beat,
> Stands every test in time and in eternity.
> It is not slow, it is not fast ;
> Its chime, its march are e'er the same ;
> Until the supreme hour has come
> It merrily goeth on.
> And when the icy hand of death
> Brings to a stop its gallant course,
> Our Lord in mercy winds it up."

In like manner he would have the following solid maxims repeated to him:

" Neither desire, nor fear, nor joy, nor suffering, nor rest, nor manifold work and employment, nor what is in me, with me, about me, nor what goes on with others, shall disturb the delightful peace of my soul; for I will seek only one thing, have to do only one thing; that is to say, the most holy will of God. Like a child on the knees of its loving mother, so will I rest in the arms of my heavenly Father."

No sufferings whatever were able to rob him of

the serenity of his soul. He knew and recognized the nearness of his death, but he was not afraid: he was reposing in the merciful arms of his heavenly Father as a child on the knees of its loving mother.

On October 16th the end of his sufferings appeared to be near at hand. Lifting up his eyes to heaven, he exclaimed: " Jesus, give me more suffering, give me more suffering ! " On the following night those around him, thinking the agony had begun, asked him if he would not receive once more the Holy Eucharist. " Of course, of course ! " he replied. " Through all my life I have prayed to have the grace of receiving Jesus in my last hour. Let my confessor come at once." During this interval he went to meet the Blessed Sacrament by yearning desires, frequently repeating the words: " Alas ! is my Saviour not come yet ? I shall die without having received Him." Dr. Kellermann came to give the beloved bishop for the last time the manna of heaven, thus to strengthen him for his passage into eternity.

Now he had no earthly wish left, and seemed as though he belonged already to heaven. " Mary, help ! St. Joseph, help ! " would he repeatedly pray. Often, too, he was heard to pronounce the name of the late Overberg, his dear friend. At various times he kissed the crucifix and the picture of Our Lady with tender devotion. So the pious sufferer lay until Sunday, October 19th. On the morning of this day his features were stamped with the signs of death. His confessor, when called, did not leave his side until the end. "Lord Jesus, Lord Jesus, do not judge me! I believe in Thee! Thou art truly the Son of God! *Miserere mei secundum magnam misericordiam Tuam!*" Such were the pious aspirations with the help of which he fought the last combat. Then he exclaimed with all the strength of his dying tongue: "Lord Jesus, come, come quickly!" "And he saith: Surely, I come quickly" (Apoc. xxii. 20). He came, and Clement Augustus, the great champion of the liberty of the Church, fell asleep in the Lord.

In May, 1852, *Cardinal Melchior von Diepenbrock*, at the suggestion of his physician, took leave of his residence in Breslau, never more to re-enter it. In August he could no longer walk up and down his room, spending most of the day reclining on a couch. But in the beginning of October the illness had so far advanced that he could not quit his bed. There he lay in pain without a complaint, without a word of impatience or apprehension. Being told that public prayers were made throughout the diocese for his recovery, and that fervent supplications rose each day to heaven, his eyes filled with tears. "God will do what is best," said he; "let His holy will be done." He loved to be alone. And when remonstrances were made to him on this account, he said: "I am not alone; the Lord is with me, and in His sweet presence it is easier to bear pain." He frequently received holy communion, and it was evident that his thoughts were beyond the earth and the things of the earth. When on the 16th of January symptoms of approaching death became manifest, he asked the young physician attending him if there was any danger. The question being answered in the affirmative, the cardinal with great composure asked for the last sacraments, and received them with a devotion which deeply moved all those around him, leaving indelible impressions on their hearts. One last greeting, one last farewell to his flock, his clergy, his chapter, and the last link which riveted him to this world was broken; henceforth his looks were turned to heaven only. The unspeakable desire of death was imprinted on his countenance; he repeatedly and fervently pressed the crucifix in his hand to his heart and lips, exclaiming: " O my Jesus, come, come ! " At midnight, the signs of approaching death growing manifest, the little household knelt round the bed of their dying bishop, who with an audible voice answered the beginning of the Litany of the Saints, " Holy Mary." This was his last word. Soon after he gently and calmly expired.